"Christianity—rightly understood—has been a tremendous inspiration and guiding star for so many in nursing. *Bioethics for Nurses* adeptly explains this past en route to laying out a Christian moral vision powerful enough to renew and sustain nursing far into the future."

– John F. Kilner
author of *Dignity and Destiny: Humanity in the Image of God*

"*Bioethics for Nurses* is very well written, and I am left with the thought, *where was this book when I was an undergrad?* The history of Christianity and how it is intertwined with the nursing profession is well documented and is clearly the underpinning of the book. The case studies and personal anecdotes from frontline nurses add credibility and an opportunity for the reader to relate."

– Michele Acito
executive vice president and chief nursing officer at
Holy Name Medical Center, Teaneck, New Jersey

"There are few vocations that imitate more directly the incarnate and transfiguring nature of Jesus Christ's love for humanity than nursing. And yet, how often does the deep connection—both historically and conceptually—between this most trusted of professions and Christian morality go unremarked upon? *Bioethics for Nurses* does more to alleviate this egregious silence in its first chapter alone than any other treatment of the topic I am familiar with, all while remaining clear, engaging, and persuasive. As an educator who works for a faith-based health sciences institution, I greatly appreciated this treatment of nursing ethics. It will serve as a beacon of hope for the future of the field and will be useful for any professor or practitioner who is tasked with furthering the healing ministry of Jesus."

– Bo Bonner
director of the Center for Human Flourishing at
Mercy College of Health Sciences

BIOETHICS FOR NURSES

A Christian Moral Vision

Alisha N. Mack, DNP, RN, FNP-C
Charles C. Camosy, PhD

William B. Eerdmans Publishing Company
Grand Rapids, Michigan

Wm. B. Eerdmans Publishing Co.
4035 Park East Court SE, Grand Rapids, Michigan 49546
www.eerdmans.com

Published 2022
Printed in the United States of America

28 27 26 25 24 23 22   1 2 3 4 5 6 7

ISBN 978-0-8028-7892-2

Library of Congress Cataloging-in-Publication Data

A catalog record for this book is available from the Library of Congress.

Biblical quotations marked (KJV) are from the King James Version. Biblical quotations marked (NIV) are from the New International Version. Biblical quotations marked (NLT) are from the New Living Translation. Biblical quotations marked (NRSV) are from the New Revised Standard Version.

In addition to the nurses who are fighting the good fight every day, I would like to dedicate this book to my grandfather. His love and support impacted me more than he will ever know. Thank you for showing me the world is kind and that love always wins.

Alisha

I dedicate this book to the nurses and nursing aids who have worked the frontlines of the COVID-19 pandemic. In risking their lives selflessly for the human dignity of their vulnerable patients—even when hope for survival was lost—they stirred up the echoes of the nurses of old.

Charlie

CONTENTS

ACKNOWLEDGMENTS

In a strange way, though we (Alisha and Charlie) both had several children to parent during a pandemic that was incredibly hard on them (and us) in multiple ways, nevertheless we both agreed that it was an appropriate time to be writing a book like this. Indeed, some of the cases we ended up using as examples were unfolding in real time as we were writing! For all of the COVID-19 pandemic's tragedy and death, perhaps there was never a better time to fully appreciate what nurses bring to our healthcare system—and American culture at large—particularly when it comes to caring for the whole person.

We have known each other a long time (chapter 1 gets a bit more into this story), but we independently came to the conclusion that not enough attention was being paid to nursing bioethics in general—and that there is virtually no attention paid to nursing bioethics for Christians in particular. Especially since bioethics often suffers from either (1) being largely unaware of clinical realities or (2) being largely unaware of academic ethics, we decided to merge our respective backgrounds as coauthors to create a book that not only filled this huge gap, but did so in a way that was both ethically serious and clinically aware.

And here that book is! We wish to sincerely and profusely thank James Ernest and Eerdmans for giving us the opportunity to write it—even in the midst of a pandemic that was so hard on so many.

Charlie wishes to single out for special thanks his primary research assistant for this book, Mary Bedway, who (among other things) did literature search after endless literature search for us. Two other research assistants, Henry Omeike and Carlton Chase, also made significant contributions to the project. Charlie especially wants to thank Bo Bonner, Director of the Center for Human Flourishing and Mercy College of Health Sciences, who generously hosted a book manuscript symposium from which we received important feedback from a wide variety of thoughtful reviewers: from doctors to doulas! He also wishes to thank a number of people who helped at various stages of the project by answering a particular question or giving overall feedback on what we were planning to do: Brother Ignatius, Carly Ann, Tita Cristie, Alfred, Mary, and Jeffery.

Alisha wants to give a special thanks to her husband (Ken) and four children (Taylor, Ellie, Isaiah, and Logan). They have been a huge support to her during the entire process. She would like to thank the many people who have shown her what good patient care looks like: the devoted nurses she has worked with over the years, the dedicated physicians, her collaborating physician Brandon, her fellow advanced practice nurses, and the faculty she has had the privilege teaching alongside. She also wants to thank the nursing faculty at Indiana Wesleyan University for providing rich feedback and support during the writing process. She could not go without thanking her nursing students, who inspire her every day. And Alisha would like to give a special thanks to the many patients she has had the privilege of taking care of, who have impacted her life and calling in more ways than she can express.

INTRODUCTION

Why a book on Christian bioethics for nurses? First, because there are many millions of nurses around the world and in the United States who identify as Christian. Second, because it is impossible to understand even what medicine is apart from deeply held beliefs and values, and it is extremely difficult for many Christian nurses to separate their vocation as a nurse from their calling as a Christian. Indeed, for many millions of nurses (particularly for Christians raised outside the secular West), this kind of separation is virtually impossible. Third, the overwhelming majority of bioethics books are focused on doctoring, not nursing. Remarkably, no bioethics book exists specifically for the millions of nurses and nursing students who identify as Christian. Though many different kinds of people may be interested in engaging the topics we cover in this book, we write it primarily for Christian nurses.

The numbers of religious people in nursing professions are staggering. According to the World Health Organization, there are over twenty million nurses or midwives globally.[1] Pew research finds that about 84 percent of the world's population identifies with an organized religion, so we can very roughly estimate that somewhere around fifteen million nurses and midwives are explicitly religious. Since about 30 percent of the world population identifies as Christian, we can also very roughly estimate that there are about six million nurses who identify explicitly with the world's largest religion. And in part, because religious people around the world tend to be younger and have more children than those who do not identify as religious, this kind of religiosity is expected to grow globally, not decline, in the decades to come.[2]

The numbers will vary in different contexts, of course, including from country to country. In the United States, there are about four million registered nurses and 300,000 nurse practitioners.[3] And during the decade 2016–2026, the US government expects the country to add 200,000 new registered nurse positions.[4] Despite a slide away from formal church membership in some contexts,[5] the US is still disproportionately religious compared to other rich Western countries: about seven in ten identify as Christian, with about 25 percent identifying as evangelical Protestant and about 20 percent identifying as Catholic.[6] Very roughly speaking, this means that there are about three million Christian nurses and nurse practitioners in the United States, with a bit over one million identifying as evangelical Protestant and a bit under one million identifying as Catholic.

The United States overall, though still very religious by the standards of most developed Western countries, is trending somewhat more secular—especially among those who are younger, male, and white.[7] This trend, however, should be weighed against a nursing profession in the United States heavily influenced by female immigrants of color—particularly female immigrants of color coming from places much more religious than the United States. According to analysis from the *Journal of the American Medical Association*, one in four nurses and home health aides in the US (over one million people) were born outside the United States.[8] Eight in ten immigrant nurses come from somewhere other than Europe or Canada. Many of these immigrant nurses are coming from deeply Christian areas like Mexico, Central and South America, the Caribbean, Africa, and Asia (particularly from countries like the Philippines).[9]

These facts about the US nursing population balance out any broader shift against religion (that is, particularly among white young men). Nurses in the United States are, as a group, broadly religious and will remain so for the foreseeable future. Indeed, many simply cannot separate their vocational call to be a nurse from their particular call from Christ in their life more broadly. A qualitative study from the *Journal of Christian Nursing* found that several qualities of Christian nurses were different from the qualities of nurses not motivated by religion—including "reliance on God for strength, the permeating work of prayer, and sense of being God's ambassador." Also important for these nurses was that what they did produced results "that matter for eternity."[10] These nurses are committed to embodying the gospel of Jesus Christ and (especially for Catholic Christians) the tradition and teaching of the Church in ways that cannot be relegated to their personal or private lives. Instead, their faith demands that they practice nursing a certain way. After all, it was their faith which led them to be nurses in the first place.

Especially given the explosion of bioethics books and articles since the 1970s, it is at least very odd that millions and millions of Christian nurses and nursing students could not—until now—read a bioethics book that was written for them specifically as Christians. This can be explained at least in part by a secular cultural shift in US medicine. Just as bioethics was coming into its own, US medicine as a profession was trying to separate itself from religion. And at this point, it is fair to say, this separation has been largely accomplished. In fact, Alisha's story of how she came to her current religious and professional place maps very well onto this topic.

ALISHA'S STORY

Alisha's nursing career started like many things God has called her to do: that is, it began before she even knew it was happening. At age fifteen, her first real job was working as a dietary aide in a nursing home—the only available job in her small town at the time. The job came at a time when she was feeling a pull toward God and began attending her local church to learn more about Christianity. After several months of working as a dietary aide, the nursing home director offered to pay for her to become certified as a nursing assistant. Alisha's new role included feeding, bathing, dressing, and caring for the residents. She loved the ability to connect with the residents by providing these basic care needs. It soon became clear that there was no other profession that would allow her to do the work of Jesus Christ quite like nursing did.

At seventeen, Alisha had the life-changing experience of working as a nursing assistant at a Catholic hospital. She saw nurses praying with their patients. She worked in a hospital where there were Bible verses written on the walls. The hospital partnered with local ministries to help provide care to those who were underserved or unable to pay. The staff she worked with were primarily Christian and their ministry was very apparent to their patients. Through this experience, Alisha felt her calling crystallize: she was to become a nurse. She worked in this role for several years before going on to become a family nurse practitioner.

Throughout her career thus far, she has worked in several different areas of specialization, including a pediatric unit, a medical/surgical unit, and a few different outpatient clinics. Her first job as a family nurse practitioner was at a local homeless shelter, where she cared for the residents and others in the community who were economically disadvantaged. The patients there were desperate for hope and for someone to validate their importance. That position allowed Alisha to openly share her faith and talk to patients about God, but she later worked at other clinics where this was discouraged. The majority of her nursing experience was working in more secular settings where faith was not openly discussed with patients outside of the broad, generic discussion of the importance of spiritual health. It was very clear that a big part of her ministry was missing.

God eventually opened the door for Alisha to step into the world of teaching. Her first teaching job was at a public university where education and religion are firmly separated from each other. This was a fundamental challenge for Alisha. Throughout her entire nursing profession, she has always seen nursing as a ministry. How could she separate the teaching of skills and knowledge from the calling and ministry of nursing? How could she teach about the history or ethics of nursing while checking religion at the door? Alisha found that, even at a public university, many of her students were Christian. While a good number of her students chose nursing for reasons other than a spiritual calling, there were still a large number of people going into nursing because they, like Alisha herself, felt called by God to the profession. She now works for a nursing school that is explicitly Christian and feels right at home being able to be fully engaged as a Christian as she trains new students in the field.

CHARLIE'S STORY

Charlie's experience was similar to that of Alisha's. Alisha struggled to express herself as a Christian nurse and nurse practitioner; Charlie's struggle came in the academic field of bioethics. Charlie grew up a cradle Catholic in very rural Wisconsin. He could walk to the local country church from his house. He was very religious as a young boy, even going to serve weekday mass in the summer when there would only be three or four people in the congregation.

He eventually grew to appreciate the close relationship between faith and reason as a philosophy major and master's student in theology at Notre Dame. As a theology teacher at a Catholic high school just outside of Milwaukee, Charlie taught a course to juniors called "Social Justice and Medical Ethics" and fell in love with the topic. The gospel of Jesus Christ made no artificial distinction between these two fields. Nor did it break down into "conservative" or "progressive" points of view. The gospel claims our whole selves as believers in ways that US political and academic categories cannot express or contain. We are called to love one another as Christ loves us: unconditionally and with a special preference for those who are vulnerable and hurting wherever we find them. This is true whether we find them on the border of our country, in the womb, on the street, on death row, or in hospitals and clinics.

After three years teaching high school, Charlie decided to study social justice and medical ethics at a higher level and went back to get his doctorate in moral theology at Notre Dame. He felt blessed to study at a place with great mentors, colleagues, and friends who were also committed to the gospel in ways which resisted the right vs. left, conservative vs. progressive binaries. During his doctoral studies, Charlie taught a bioethics course for nurses at Indiana University-South Bend and met his coauthor, Alisha (who was easily the best student in his class). Once he got his first job as a full-time professor, however, and started attending professional academic conferences, he realized just how different the rest of the bioethics field was from his previous experiences. Bioethics tended to make very hard distinctions between conservative and progressive, faith and reason.

We will focus in detail on this topic in chapter 3, but the more time Charlie spent in the field of bioethics the more he realized that his religious views were simply not welcome—especially (although not only) if they were deemed to be "conservative" by his secular colleagues. One could attend all the formal sessions of the field's most important annual conference—put on by the American Society of Bioethics and Humanities—and never hear a paper delivered which explicitly invoked faith or theology as a key part of the argument. This despite the fact that Christian theologians invented the field and were, in fact, the first bioethicists![11] Traditions of secular moral thought—even if shared only by a small minority of people, and even if they directly contradict the dominant secular traditions—are welcomed into today's bioethics conversation. But traditions of Christian moral thought are most often pushed to the margins. Today, Charlie teaches theology and bioethics in a Jesuit-Catholic theology department and writes books and articles for both Christians and those who are genuinely open-minded and committed to viewpoint diversity.

OUR GOALS FOR THIS BOOK

Alisha's and Charlie's stories illustrate a structural problem with medicine and bioethics today: these fields are most often organized in a way which is unfriendly—and sometimes even hostile—to those who want to practice medicine and/or bioethics on the basis of their explicit religious faith. In this larger context, it may seem less odd that there are no bioethics books designed for the millions of Christian nurses. There is a focus on doctoring over nursing (a bias we will address in chapter 2) that helps explain this void in part, yet there are several secular books on nursing bioethics. That there are no Christian theological books on nursing bioethics is best explained by the hyper-secular culture of a field that often makes such approaches unwelcome.

In light of this massive gap, we write this book (while of course in conversation with secular and other non-Christian thinkers and practitioners) from an explicitly theological perspective as committed Christians ourselves. We want to speak directly to Christian nurses and advanced practice nurses and Christians studying to work in these fields. We start with the foundational claim that even coming to a coherent idea of what the practice of medicine is in the first place (to say nothing of dealing with hard ethical questions in practice) requires drawing on one's deepest and most foundational views about what is ultimately true. That is, it requires drawing on one's theological beliefs.

We both want to emphasize that being a Christ follower means rejecting the idea that one belongs to the so-called right or left. Indeed, we write this book for Christians from all over the political spectrum. Alisha is an evangelical Christian and Charlie is a Catholic Christian, and this means there will be some differences in our approach, but our goal is to speak the truth in love to each other and to our readers. We also wrote a book that—in addition to being used in the classroom at colleges and universities with mission-centered nursing programs—can benefit current nurses or advanced practice nurses, including nurse practitioners, clinical nurse specialists, nurse anesthetists, and nurse midwives. Nursing can sometimes be a lonely and frustrating field for those who are driven by their faith. We hope this book can both remind you that you are not alone and offer resources for feeling more grounded and confident in refusing to choose between your faith and your profession.

HOW THIS BOOK WILL PROCEED

The biases in medicine and bioethics described above have created a number of influential myths, and the first section of our book will attempt to bust three significant ones. In chapter 1, we challenge the oft-repeated claim that "nursing began" with Florence Nightingale by focusing on the explicitly Christian roots of the profession, particularly among the Sisters of Mercy in Ireland. In chapter 2 we build on contemporary challenges to the idea that doctoring is somehow more important than or prior to nursing by, again, focusing on history which suggests something quite different. We also present a vision of nursing that is very much in line with current trends in medicine—especially a focus on the whole person and social determinants of health. In chapter 3 we bust some of the myths that lead those in power to push theology and faith away from the practice of medicine and bioethics.

Chapter 4 draws on the insights of the three previous chapters to make a case for our common Christian theological ideas and principles to shape our vision of nursing. The second part of our book will lay out a Christian bioethical vision for nursing in the real world. Chapters 5 through 11 will put this vision and these principles into action by showing how they function in several case studies that both illustrate the importance and implications of the principles, and also help current and future nurses and advanced practice nurses prepare for similar or analogous situations that they may one day face themselves.

Finally, the third part of the book focuses on the future of nursing, clearly a "profession on the move." Chapter 12 focuses in particular on why it is so important for nurses to have their consciences protected—not only because of basic human rights—but because Christianity requires that we love God with everything that we are. Chapter 13 focuses on nurses taking their rightful place on medicine teams, especially in light of the fact that nursing is at the forefront of exciting movements in medicine, like patient- and relationship-centered care, care of the whole person, and social determinants of health. And finally, in Chapter 14 we explore what nursing looked like during the COVID-19 pandemic and how this will change the process moving into the future.

Now, however, let us turn to myth busting. And let us begin with the myths surrounding the very ideas about how nursing began.

PART ONE

Recovering a Nursing Vision

1

THE CHRISTIAN ORIGINS OF CONTEMPORARY NURSING

> It is such a blessing to have been called, however unworthy, to be the handmaid of the Lord.
>
> – *Florence Nightingale*

The popular imagination often thinks of the practice of Western health care as secular. Maybe even hyper-secular. Religion and science "don't mix" in the minds of many influential people in medicine. But this view is difficult to reconcile with history. As with most institutions in the developed Western world, our health-care practices come directly out of an explicitly Christian culture and from explicitly Christian ideals and practices. This is true when we look at the history of hospitals, when we look at the history of doctoring, and especially when we look at the history of nursing.

But wait, aren't nursing students taught that nursing begins with a data-driven, secular pioneer named Florence Nightingale? This is an important myth to bust early in this book, and for two reasons. First, Florence Nightingale was anything but secular. As Mary Sullivan points out in her book on Nightingale's correspondence with Mother Mary Clare Moore of the Sisters of Mercy, this nursing pioneer "was deeply engaged in the religious and philosophical thought of her time and that the primary aim of her life was not to reform social institutions but to serve God."[1] Indeed, her calling as a nurse no doubt has much in common with many of those reading this book. Second, as is made clear through her relationship with the Sisters of Mercy and other religious orders, Nightingale was learning from and building upon an already well-established Christian foundation for the practice of nursing. As significant as she was for the development of nursing today, the practice predates Nightingale by hundreds of years.

We will explore more about why this is the case in chapter 3, but one frustrating aspect of many contemporary discussions of Western-style health care is the near erasure of its Christian historical foundations. Especially given the primary audience we have in mind for this book, but also for those who simply want an authentic understanding of how nursing came to be what it is today, we are actively working against the erasure of this history. To that end, we will begin this chapter by focusing on the Christian origins of Western health care more broadly, and then pivot to the development of Christian nursing especially as a practice of women religious. Finally, we will show how women religious deeply influenced Florence Nightingale—and, by extension, what nursing would become after her.

CHRISTIAN ORIGINS OF WESTERN HEALTH CARE

In Charlie's previous book, which was on the relationship between contemporary secular medicine and losing our sense that all human beings are fundamentally equal, he also shows how much of our modern understanding of health care comes explicitly out of a Christian context.[2] We will say more about this in chapter 4, but one major reason Christianity had such a focus on health and healing was because this was such a priority for Christ himself. The following passage, Matthew 11:2–5, is just one of dozens of relevant examples we could have cited from the Gospels:

> When John the Baptist heard in prison what the Christ was doing, he sent word by his disciples and said to him, "Are you the one who is to come, or are we to wait for another?" Jesus answered them, "Go and tell John what you hear and see: the blind receive their sight, the lame walk, the lepers are cleansed, the deaf hear, the dead are raised, and the poor have good news brought to them." (NRSV)

When Jesus was pressed by the disciples of John the Baptist to give an account of himself so they could determine whether or not he was the Messiah, the chosen one of God, he did not speak of violent revolutions wrought by his great power. Nor did he speak of political change or invoke a regal status. Instead, he focused on the fact that sick people came to him for help—and were made whole. It is no accident that one of Jesus's most important monikers is "the Great Physician," for he directly and analogously thought of his work in precisely these terms. Significantly, Jesus often explicitly connected the physical health of a person with their spiritual health and tried to address the fullness of the needy person in front of him.

The early church, unsurprisingly, took its cues from Jesus the Great Physician by putting care of the sick and disabled, especially the untouchable sick and disabled who were discarded by the dominant culture, at the center of its ministry. Rodney Stark, Distinguished Professor of the Social Sciences at Baylor University, has argued this kind of care contributed significantly to the improbable growth of a small religious sect into what would become the official religion of the Roman Empire. Stark argues that care for (and even adoption of) the sick, disabled, and female infants who were typically exposed and left for dead (or, at best, slavery/prostitution), along with a refusal to abandon the sick during plagues, were significant factors in making the Christian witness deeply attractive to converts.[3] His research, for instance, found that after the Antonine plague (second century), the Cyprian plague (third century), and the Justinian plague (sixth century) there were significantly higher conversion rates to Christianity.

The houses of bishops and other wealthy/important Christians in the early Church were expected to be houses of hospitality for the sick. Eventually these would develop into formal hospital and nursing facilities, especially when Christianity become an accepted practice in the fourth century. There was a dramatic early instance of this in the work of Saint Ephrem who, during a plague at Edessa in 375, provided hundreds of beds for the afflicted. But perhaps the most famous early example of a hospital was that of Saint Basil at Caesarea in Cappadocia in 369. It "took on the dimensions of a city": boasting organized systems of regular streets, buildings for different kinds of patients, and even living spaces for health-care providers.[4]

The Rule of Saint Benedict, written in the early fifth century, insisted that "care of the sick is to be placed above and before every other duty."[5] The research of Andrew Crislip shows that many of these monasteries focused so intensely on health care that they eventually and naturally became full-time hospitals.[6] This set of values and practices for those who follow Jesus would prove to be deeply influential for the Christendom of the Middle Ages, which saw a dramatic increase in the numbers of hospitals and also schools for the training of health-care providers. Driven by a parallel increase in the founding of religious and military orders devoted to ministering to the sick, by the late Middle Ages "nearly every city" in Europe had what was called a "Hospital of the Holy Ghost" that was run (either in fact or in spirit) by the Order of the Hospitallers of the Holy Ghost.[7]

CHRISTIAN RELIGIOUS ORDERS AND THE FIRST NURSES

Though the contemporary distinction between nurses and doctors was not as stark as it is today, the monks and nuns who founded and ran the hospitals of the ancient and medieval worlds mentioned above were much more like what we might think of as nurses, caring for the fullness of the whole person (as Jesus Christ did), than like specialized doctors focusing on physical systems of organic plumbing. For instance, the Hospitallers of the Holy Ghost were often religious monks or nuns who took vows from the Rule of Saint Augustine—with a dual focus on the "corporal works of mercy" (which include things like caring for the sick, offering hospitality to strangers, and burying the dead) and the "spiritual works of mercy" (which include things like comforting the afflicted, praying for others, and counseling the doubtful).

By the end of the Middle Ages, and into the early modern period, orders of sister-nurses were very well established and spread throughout Europe. The Daughters of the Holy Spirit, for instance, was an important order of women religious that was founded in 1706 "to serve God by serving the poor, the sick, and the children."[8] Care for the fullness of the needs of the people they served didn't keep them from delivering excellent and thorough medical care. Indeed, especially if they were being sent to minister in rural settings where they weren't seen as competition for doctors, these sister-nurses would be trained in their mother house to practice a wide variety of medicine. Research done by Tim McHugh on this order's work in rural France, for instance, found that they were taught "to diagnose, to prescribe treatment, and to prepare medications." From the records of contracts that still exist to this day, we learn that these nuns considered "active medical intervention through the providing of remedies or through the services commonly offered by surgeons of equal importance as their nursing and spiritual consoling of the sick."[9]

Another very significant group of sister-nurses were the Daughters of Charity of St. Vincent de Paul. In the mid-1800s, Sister Mathilde Coskery wrote the first comprehensive document on nursing, which she called *Advices on Care of the Sick*. Significantly, these sisters saw their role as not only bringing physical healing to their patients, but spiritual healing as well. Indeed, Mother Mary Xavier Clark said that their patient should be able to say, when a sister leaves his bedside, "That Sister is more like an angel than a human being. The very sight of her makes me think of God and love him."[10] And though they had a focus on the spiritual, like the Daughters of the Holy Spirit before them, the Daughters of Charity were also expert in the practice of caring for the physical bodies of their patients. Florence Nightingale's encounter with a nursing mission run by the Daughters of Charity in Alexandria, Egypt, was deeply influential on her own journey toward nursing (significant for our discussion below).

The French revolution—and succeeding secular and anti-Catholic trends of the Enlightenment—encouraged the Daughters of the Holy Spirit and the Daughters of Charity to take up residence in the United States where they were afforded religious freedom to pursue their ministry.[11] They would join several other orders of women religious who focused on nursing and health care in the US, including the Sisters of Mercy, another group of sister-nurses who would have a profound influence on Florence Nightingale.

THE SISTERS OF MERCY

The Sisters of Mercy were founded in 1831 by Catherine McAuley in a poverty- and epidemic-stricken Dublin, Ireland. She explicitly focused the order's contemplative and spiritual life into direct service to the poor and marginalized, particularly homeless girls and women. Especially as they saw the infuriatingly strong connections between poverty and illness, they would soon adopt a particular focus on health care, one that would blossom into a philosophy they would call "careful nursing." This philosophy was built by McAuley directly out of her sense of Jesus Christ's "great tenderness for the sick."[12] Indeed, their commitment to having "great tenderness in all things" was at the heart of the

Sisters of Mercy motivation for moving into nursing in the first place. Their first goal in caring for any patient—at least when death as not an imminent risk—was to relieve, as best they could, whatever was causing their patient's distress. Again, the fullness of the good of the person in front of them was at the heart of how they ministered to their patients' needs.

Nurses with the Sisters of Mercy gained a reputation for having "unconditional patience, generosity, kindness and compassion towards patients and one another. This was understood to encompass a calm manner and respect for inherent human dignity."[13] Eventually, they would come to specify a general philosophy of careful nursing into specific principles and practices. Here are a few of the most important ones:[14]

- *Contagious calmness.* Quiet self-confidence exuded from these sisters as they went about their nursing tasks. Their gentle and tender manner reflected an inner calm and peace that would be further reflected in their communal environment more generally and to the patient specifically.
- *Disinterested love.* The Sisters of Mercy insisted on loving everyone—including each other, but especially their patients—based on their common relationship with God. The "disinterested" adjective here refers to an intentionally unbiased and impartial love to each person, regardless of their characteristics.
- *"Perfect" skill development.* Nursing was a kind of art for the Sisters of Mercy, but it was also very much a skilled craft to be honed and perfected. It involved close and continual observation of their patients, with meticulous attention to detail and lightning-quick responses to their needs. Particular focus was given to patients who were dying to ensure that they received every possible comfort and consolation.
- *Self-care.* In part because the job of a nurse is so difficult, especially when connected to the sufferings and deaths of so many

patients, the Sisters of Mercy insisted on a robust self-care program. This included an insistence on eating the best foods available, getting plenty of rest and exercise, and making time for social and recreational activities. In addition to maintaining an inner sense of calm and disinterested love, part of their understanding of self-care involved encouraging nurses to have a sense of humor and quick wit—with their patients, yes, but also with each other.

- *Power from service.* Jesus Christ inverted typical power dynamics. You want to be first? Put others before you. You want power? Die to self and embrace your weakness. You want glory? Embrace humility and even humiliation. The Sisters of Mercy knew that any authentic power they had came from putting the love of the marginalized ahead of their personal interests.

As we will see below, when these Sisters were called on to serve under the leadership of Florence Nightingale during the Crimean War, they immediately moved to do their work in the background willingly and without complaint. Despite this less visible role, and despite having three strikes against them (being women, Catholic, and Irish), the Sisters of Mercy ended up playing pivotal roles in almost every significant crisis Nightingale faced. They developed a sterling reputation for responding immediately, calmly, and effectively.

Florence Nightingale had a particularly transformative relationship with Mother Mary Clare Moore, who was an important partner to Catherine McAuley. We will now examine the lasting impact their relationship had on the origins of contemporary nursing.

MOTHER MARY CLARE MOORE AND FLORENCE NIGHTINGALE

Mary Clare Moore worked most closely with Catherine McCauley in coming up with The Rule and Constitutions for the Sisters of

Mercy. Though also born Irish, Moore was assigned by McCauley to be the first Mother Superior of their new convent in London. For thirty-five years she oversaw the multifaceted work of these sisters: visiting the sick poor both at home and in the hospital, instructing both children and adults in religious education, conducting school for the poor (and especially for poor girls), and providing general "material help and spiritual consolation" for the poor in "countless other ways."[15] During her time in London, Moore would found eight additional convents for her order—and even build a new hospital, St. Elizabeth's Hospital for the Incurables (the first Catholic hospital in London since the Reformation).[16] Fifteen years after starting the London community, Moore was asked by her bishop to temporarily leave her ministry in London in order to answer a desperate plea from the British government for nurses to serve the wounded of the Crimean War. She went with four of her sisters, and it was there that she met and served under Florence Nightingale.

Nightingale had first learned about nursing from the Sisters of Charity in Alexandria, Dublin, and Paris.[17] On the basis of those experiences, she was already eager to engage and learn more from this new group of sister-nurses. Indeed, during her time with the Sisters of Mercy she regularly took notes on their careful nursing practices.[18] According to Sullivan, Nightingale's personal struggles with Sisters of Mercy from a different community have been highlighted by biographers who wish to downplay the influence of religion on her thought and her life. But she was close with the sisters in Moore's community, and especially with Moore herself. Indeed, we can learn about their relationship from the numerous letters sent between them. Sullivan writes: "[Nightingale and Moore were] bound together by their devotion to the neglected, by nursing and other skills they had learned the hard way, by mature Christian faith, and by their lively affection for one another, born of mutual respect and ease of communication. It is little wonder, then, that when Clare lay dying on December

12th 1874, Florence wrote: 'It is we who are left motherless when she goes.'"[19] Despite serving under Nightingale during the war, Moore had a profound and sustaining effect on her friend—with Nightingale later saying, "I have kept all your dear letters. And you cannot think how much they have encouraged me. They are almost the only earthly encouragement I have."[20]

We will get to the spiritual influence that Moore had on Nightingale in a moment, but here it is worth highlighting the deep respect the latter had for the former when it came to the business of nursing the soldiers. In letters to Moore, Nightingale said the following:[21]

> Your going home is the greatest blow I have had yet. . . . You were far above me in fitness for the General Superintendency, both in worldly talent of administration, & far more in spiritual qualifications from which God values in a superior. . . . What you have done for the work no one can ever say.

And:

> I always felt you ought to have been the Superior & I the inferior. . . . I always felt how magnanimous your spiritual obedience in taking up such a position . . . & how I should have failed without your help. . . . I always wondered at your unfailing patience, sweetness, forbearance, and courage under the many trials peculiar to yourselves, beyond what was common to all.

Perhaps even more important than this, however, was the effect that Mary Clare Moore had on her friend's spiritual life. Nightingale, like many of us, went through different stages in her spiritual life, but her continued contact with Moore after the war, especially in their exchange of spiritual and theological books, helped her become what Sullivan calls a "mature Christian." Both believed that true Christian faith was found in doing good work on behalf of the marginalized, and not "simply or primarily in private expressions of religious faith."[22] But they also both understood (and Nightingale developed this view more strongly as her friendship with Moore unfolded) that the spiritual basis had to be there as a foundation. They had a "common desire for purity of heart" in ways that helped them consistently recognize that what they were trying to do "rested wholly on God."[23] Nightingale said Moore never tried to convert her to Catholicism, but she nevertheless recognized just how powerfully present God was in this Mother Superior's life. Indeed, when she wrote one of Moore's fellow sisters to inquire about her friend's failing health, she said of Moore, "Perhaps she is at this moment with God. But this we know: She could scarcely be more with God than she was habitually here."[24]

There were times Nightingale was more disparaging of traditional Christianity. But the historical evidence shows that Moore's influence on her friend was instrumental to her developing a mature Christian faith. According to Sullivan, the "central reason for their twenty-year friendship" was their common "dedication to life-affirming work undertaken and pursued in fidelity to what they perceived to be God's will."[25] In one letter, Nightingale invokes Saint Theresa and says "it is *such* a blessing to have been called, however unworthy, to be the 'handmaid of the Lord [emphasis original].'" In another she explains her view that "Christ on the Cross" is the "highest expression" of God and that God hangs on the cross every day in each one of us.[26] The primary aim of Florence Nightingale's life was not, Sullivan insists, to reform wretched conditions, but rather to love God well.

TO THE UNITED STATES AND OUR CONTEMPORARY MOMENT

As Europe became less and less welcoming to religious orders, many of them moved their work to places like the United States.

Only thirty years after their founding, the Sisters of Mercy were tending to the wounded of the US Civil War and were publicly and lavishly praised by President Abraham Lincoln for doing so.[27] He was right to offer such praise, for he had virtually nowhere else to turn: at the start of the war Catholic nuns were the only trained nurses available.[28] The Sisters of Mercy and Daughters of Charity were among a dozen religious orders who served.

To give one more example, the US Navy formally recognized that the Sisters of the Holy Cross were the first members of the Navy Nursing Corps given their work ferrying wounded soldiers up the Ohio River. As Nightingale had similarly discovered just a few years earlier, Secretary of War Edwin Stanton found that these religious orders were invaluable for organizing health care delivery quickly and expertly. Just before the Civil War, religious orders already ran twenty-eight US hospitals and Stanton and other leaders sought them out to run and serve in Union military hospitals as well. These religious orders would go on to found approximately 220 nursing schools by 1915. And, in so doing, they "stamped their distinct understanding of nursing onto secular society."[29] Many of these schools still exist and are flourishing to this day.[30] In addition to administering hospitals and schools, contemporary women religious orders are still doing direct work for the most vulnerable in health-care fields. Indeed, many US nuns gave selfless service to the elderly and disabled in nursing homes during the COVID-19 pandemic.[31]

It is fair to say, however, that nursing in the United States overall ended up straying from its religious roots in the late nineteenth and early twentieth centuries. Indeed—and in our view this is no accident—nursing in the US has also largely lost this older vision of itself as having a role of leadership to play in health care, rightly along with physicians. This has been changing in the last decade or so, though, and it is to these trends and questions we now turn.

DISCUSSION QUESTIONS

1. The Rule of Saint Benedict insists that "care of the sick is to be placed above and before every other duty." How does this claim align with what is written in Scripture?
2. Reflect on the Sisters of Mercy's principles and practices for careful nursing: contagious calmness, disinterested love, perfect skill development, self-care, and power from service. Which one(s) are hardest to put into practice? What are the barriers for doing so?
3. We examined the spiritual influence that Mother Mary Clare Moore had on Florence Nightingale. What spiritual influence can you have on your fellow nursing colleagues? How can we better support each other in the vocation?

2

THE SHIFTING ROLE OF THE NURSE

> The trained nurse has become one of the great blessings of humanity, taking a place beside the physician and the priest.
>
> – *Dr. William Osler*

In this chapter, we turn our focus to the role of the nurse. What is a nurse? Who gets to define nursing? While the particular duties of nurses have of necessity changed across the centuries, the foundational role of nursing has not. At the very heart of a nurse is a trained professional who seeks to provide care, comfort, and compassion to the patients she serves. Unfortunately, some have viewed nurses as secondary to "real medicine" or merely assistants to physicians. But in this chapter we will dispel this myth by highlighting the role of nurses, and the often unrecognized impact they have on the overall health of patients and communities. We will begin by giving an overview of how nurses—once considered health-care crusaders in the mold of Florence Nightingale and Sister Mary Clare Moore—became portrayed as mere assistants to physicians. We will then discuss nursing as its own profession and the importance of this profession for the care of patients in the fullness of who they are. And we would be amiss in a project like this if we did not devote a section to the Christian nurse—which is both a profession and a calling. Finally, we will discuss the current direction health care is going and the responsibility, and privilege, nurses have to lead the change.

A SHIFT IN THE ROLE OF NURSES

Before we discuss the shift in the role of nurses, it is important to remind ourselves some of what we just discussed in chapter 1: religion and medicine have had a long relationship. Throughout most of history the two were strongly interconnected, until being separated only recently. Throughout the Middle Ages the church was the main provider of care for the poor and sick. In fact, prior to the Christian era, there was nothing that we would recognize today as a hospital. The church was primarily responsible for running these hospitals and even granted licenses to physicians.[1] Nurses were very often the main providers of care, both in the physical hospitals as well as going out into the streets and bringing care to the sick.

While this setup continued for centuries, several shifts occurred that caused significant changes in how roles in health care were conceived—where medicine became the dominant force. As Michael John Pritchard puts it, "Any attempt to analyze how the medical profession became so dominant in health care, must as a starting point, understand that this dominance was not achieved overnight."[2] The main catalyst was the shift toward medicine becoming the kind of discipline that was separated from religion. By establishing medicine as this kind of discipline—with specific guidelines on training apart from the Christian church—the profession slowly gained state-sanctioned autonomy and self-regulation. This, in turn, allowed medicine to dictate a lot of health-care decisions, including who could legally treat a sick person and which professions—including nursing—would fall under medical control.[3] This gap widened even further with the predominant viewpoint on gender roles. At the time of this shift, physicians were primarily male and nurses were primarily female. So, the conditions were perfect: medicine separated from religion during a time of pre-established gender roles.

A quote taken from *The Household Physician* in 1902 paints a picture of the view of the nurse's role by physicians during this time: "A nurse must begin her work with the idea firmly implanted in her mind that she is only the instrument by whom the doctor gets his instructions carried out: she occupies no independent position in the treatment of the sick person."[4] This view continued for most of the century, and indeed still persists in some circles to this day. A few years ago, in fact, there was a front-page news article that described nurses as "assistants" to physicians in the management of patient care.[5] Fortunately, nursing has been able to slowly rise above this misrepresentation of what nurses do and the role they actually play. What nurses do and the role they play, it turns out, can and should be described as a profession.

THE PROFESSION OF NURSING

With the background of how the myth evolved firmly in our minds, let's begin busting the myth that nurses are merely assistants or handmaidens to physicians—or servants to patients and families. Nurses are educated, well-trained professionals in the science of patient care.[6] This training and experience makes the profession of nursing something that goes well beyond merely assisting physicians and following their orders. By traditional definition, nursing has fulfilled every criterion of being a profession: it has its own particular body of knowledge, code of ethics, autonomy, conducts its own research, and convenes its own regulatory and accrediting bodies.[7] As a profession, it also has its own nursing diagnosis list, which is supported by research and formulated after assessing the patient and deciding on necessary interventions to reach patient goals and improve outcomes.[8]

Nursing is centered on a relationship between the nurse and the patient, whether that is an individual, a family, or the community. Nurses provide care and assistance in order to facilitate recovery, prevent diseases, and promote wellness.[9] But most importantly, nursing is a beautiful, intricate blend of science and art. This particular blend is what makes nursing such a powerful force. It is also what makes nursing such an honored profession and ranking as the most trusted profession year after year.[10] Yes, nurses are educated in the science of the human body and, like physicians, they continue to learn and grow in this knowledge throughout their careers. Yes, they spend years mastering the science of nursing through the act of caring for patients.[11] But there is nothing about this that takes away from also understanding nursing as an art. Indeed, the kind of technical skills nurses learn blend perspective with the art of caring for patients.

Florence Nightingale understood this well. "Nursing is an art," she said. "And if it is to be made an art, it requires an exclusive devotion as hard a preparation as any painter's or sculptor's work; for what is having to do with dead canvas or dead marble, compared with having to do with the living body, the temple of God's spirit? It is one of the Fine Arts."[12] The art of nursing isn't just focused on the act of curing the physical body, as important as that is, but rather on both the act of curing *and* caring. A nurse's artful care can appear in many forms: from having the time and capacity to form a trusting relationship with one's patient, to having the ability to understand exactly what the patient is saying even if no words are ever expressed, to the act of simply being with the patient in silence and affirming that they are not alone. In many cases, the art of nursing comes in the form of intuition developed from years of experience working on the frontlines of health care.[13] Unlike the science of nursing, the practice of the nursing arts focuses on experiences and the meaning of those experiences. As one nurse beautifully stated, it helps us to "connect with patients during care and is completely reliant upon being genuine, attentive, and immersed in the moment with patients—what some call being in true presence."[14] These characteristics are often what patients remember most about the nurses who cared for them, often in their moments of greatest vulnerability and need.

THE ROLE OF THE CHRISTIAN NURSE

The shift toward nursing as a mere servant of doctor and patient, one from which nursing is happily recovering, happened when the profession strayed from its original Christian roots described in the previous chapter. This is important since a large percentage of nurses still identify as Christian and go into nursing as a spiritual ministry. For these nurses, there is another component to being a nurse, one that adds even more depth to the profession by going beyond science and art: the spiritual calling. Many nurses' fundamental skills are transformed when they are motivated by a genuinely Christian spiritual life. Alisha notes that her own experience as a Christian nurse tracks with what is documented in the *Journal of Christian Nursing*: our acts become bigger than caring and comforting and become a way for the hurting world to experience God through us.[15] And while all nurses provide care and comfort, the Christian nurse offers an additional component, something even more powerful: to be the hands and feet of Jesus and through this, to bring others closer to God. From our perspective, there is little that is more powerful than this.

Christian nurses have for many centuries looked to the Gospels as guidance for how to care for others. Jesus, who was regarded as the Great Physician, devoted much of his time to healing. Nearly a full third of the New Testament Gospels embody healing narratives.[16] This classic Scripture passage from Matthew 25:35–40 has captured the imagination of many Christian nurses as a framework for their calling:

> "For I was hungry and you gave me something to eat, I was thirsty and you gave me something to drink, I was a stranger

> and you invited me in, I needed clothes and you clothed me, I was sick and you looked after me, I was in prison and you came to visit me."
>
> Then the righteous will answer him, "Lord, when did we see you hungry and feed you, or thirsty and give you something to drink? When did we see you a stranger and invite you in, or needing clothes and clothe you? When did we see you sick or in prison and go to visit you?"
>
> The King will reply, "Truly I tell you, whatever you did for one of the least of these brothers and sisters of mine, you did for me." (NIV)

The role of the Christian nurse takes on a new meaning when we care for others as Jesus cared for them—and when we see His face in the face of our vulnerable patients, many of whom are, in fact, the "least" ones in our culture.

Even in the face of adversity and workplace challenges, the ministry of a Christian nurse's calling can provide the hope, strength, and endurance we need to continue on. Such a nurse can see past patients' behaviors and words and view them with an understanding that they are in need of care, comfort, and respect. Christian nurses can treat them knowing that their vocation is pleasing to God and their ministry mirrors that of Jesus himself. For it is Jesus who moves Christians to follow his compassionate example and heal the sick and comfort the afflicted. Those of us who are Christian nurses have a duty to follow Christ's particular example, to "go and do likewise."

We will say more about our Christian theological vision for a Christian bioethics for nurses in chapter 4. But here it does make sense to say that a love that is Christ-imitating cares for others regardless of status, gender, income, or condition. It cannot be contained by boundaries of the world. In fact, Christ often showed the most compassion for those whom the world had tossed away by busting through the cultural boundaries that keep the privileged separate from those on the margins. Countless nurses, as well as Christian physician groups, have continued this legacy, including Florence Nightingale herself who, as we saw in the previous chapter, took her faith in Christ quite seriously. Often referred to as "the lady with the lamp," Nightingale felt a calling early on to care for the poor and the sick. Throughout her years as a nurse, she treated thousands of patients, cared for wounded soldiers, opened the first nurse training school, and forever impacted epidemiology and public health. She is remembered as a nursing pioneer, Crimean War heroine, and health-care reformer.[17] She should also be remembered as a nurse who intentionally served God through her profession.

Catherine of Siena is another example—also known as a "Patroness of Nursing," she devoted her life to caring for patients who were considered the most hopeless or unfriendly and difficult and worked tirelessly to help the poor and those who were suffering. It was even cited that she walked the streets at night looking for patients in need.[18] What a picture of love and devotion for the sick and vulnerable!

It is also important to remember the impact Christianity played in the development of the US health-care system. Our hospitals were founded by religious groups, primarily Catholic sisters, to serve the poor and needy. The impact of these religious groups on the development of the American health system was immense. As Peter Levin noted, "Their historical record as founders, builders, financiers, and managers of hospitals is unmatched by any other group between 1850 and 1950. And, this was accomplished at a time when women played no similar leadership and institutional ownership role elsewhere in society."[19] In honor of these health-care pioneers, let us not forget where our health-care system originated from and not lose sight of the important role each one of us plays in the future of health-care practices. In upcoming chapters, we will dive deeper into the theological ideas and commitments of the Christian nurse, especially as they relate to the duties to care for people and what it means to love and care for patients in the fullness of who they are. Happily for Christian nurses, what that calling from God means specifically matches up very well with current trends in health care.

THE SHIFT TO WHOLE-PERSON CARE

While nursing and medicine are both essential examples of the health-care professions, and must work together for the good of today's patients, they are distinct, having been founded from two different philosophies and traditions. Traditionally, medicine has focused on healing the body through the curing of physical disease. At first, doctoring in the Western tradition had a very clear connection between the mind and the body. Even Hippocrates—known by many as the Father of Western Medicine—spoke quite clearly about the relationship between the mind and body. But Western medicine began separating itself from traditional doctoring during the Enlightenment, with particular influence coming from Descartes's influential theory of dualism in which the mind and body work as separate and distinct parts.[20] Under this model, patients were viewed as a series of parts that needed to be fixed—either through medication, surgery, or other procedure—in order to keep the body functioning at its best. While some physicians still practice with this belief system, there has been, fortunately, a much greater respect for the mind-body connection in recent years.

Nursing has walked a different historical path, as we just saw in chapter 1. The profession of nursing grew out of a Christian foundation where patients are all humans, created in the image of God, and encompasses body, mind, and spirit.[21] Nursing today, even outside of the Christian influence, still views patients through a holistic lens based on the understanding that a patient's biological, psychological, and spiritual aspects are interconnected to form a unique person and care should be individualized to each patient's diverse needs.[22] As nurse theorist Patricia Benner wrote, "Nurses deal with not only normality and pathophysiology but also with the lived social and skilled body in promoting health, growth, and development and in caring for the sick and dying."[23]

Perhaps not surprisingly given what we know about the profession, many of the early proponents of the "patient-centered" and "whole person" models of care were nurses, including advanced practice registered nurses (APRNs). The traditional model included more of a paternalistic view where the provider, who is the only expert worth consulting, made the decisions. Patients played a very small role in their own health care. Patients would almost never question a physician or request an alternative treatment; the doctor's words were accepted as final and complete.[24] Here is one example of this taken from the 1847 *Code of Medical Ethics*, published by the American Medical Association. It is taken from a section titled "Obligations of Patients to Their Physicians": "The obedience of a patient to the prescriptions of his physician should be prompt and implicit. He should never permit his own crude opinions as to their fitness, to influence his attention to them. A failure in one particular may render an otherwise judicious treatment dangerous, and even fatal."[25]

Many generations witnessed patients being treated like children and viewed as unschooled and unable to make medical-related decisions. And while there are still providers who practice with this paternalistic approach, the last few decades have witnessed a breakdown of the once-held belief that the physician is an all-knowing healer. Research has shown that shared decision-making—where patients play an active role in their care—results in improved treatment adherence, outcomes, quality of life, and disease coping.[26] Over the last several years patients have taken a more active role in their health care and desire to have a voice in their care. And as a result, health-care providers have a much wider range of data to use when thinking about how to serve the health of the whole person in front of them. And nurses, through their training as patient advocates, have been absolutely invaluable in helping patients navigate this role. And who better to assist patients with self-advocacy than the ones who spend the most time with patients, developing a deeper understanding of their needs, wants, and gaps in care? And who better to love patients in the fullness of the people God created them to be?

THE NURSE'S VOICE

Nurses make up the largest group of professionals in health care. With four million nurses in the US and counting, nurses represent the base of the pyramid, the foundation of health care itself.[27] Without nurses there would be no health-care system. Despite this, and for reasons related to some of what was just mentioned above, nurses' voices have not always been respected or requested. We should be forthright about something here: nurses' thoughts and opinions on patient care have not always been welcomed. Something similar can be said about policymakers and administrators when it comes to nurses' views for improving health-care policy and delivery.

This seems to be one of the greatest oversights in our health-care system. Nurses spend the most time with patients. Their opinions should not only be counted but should be encouraged and even become a formal process of the decision-making of the medical team. Nurses spend countless hours at the bedside caring for patients. They develop a relationship with patients and are oftentimes the voices of the patients and family members. Nurses often cultivate a kind of "sixth sense" or intuition that can be used to pick up subtle cues about a patient's status. Indeed, nurses are often the first health-care workers to detect when patients are deteriorating. In these situations, nurses become patient advocates to ensure they receive the necessary attention and care to improve their status. In fact, patient advocacy is one of the provisions in the American Nurses Association's Code of Ethics: "The nurse promotes, advocates for, and protects the rights, health, and safety of the patient."[28] But patient advocacy must be met with support from others on the health-care team. Alisha, both as a nurse as well as clinical faculty, has personally witnessed many situations in which nurses' opinions and suggestions were not taken seriously. This often resulted in compromised care. But there were also times where her concerns were respected, treatment was altered, and care for the patient improved. The provider understood her place on the team and appreciated her intuition, and this allowed for respectful collaboration and improved patient outcomes.

Nurses are also the liaison between the health-care provider and patient in respect to the patient's treatment plan. When a patient is unable to follow through with a provider's treatment recommendations, it is often the nurse who speaks up. And how often are patients being labeled "noncompliant," when in reality, there are factors in play that go beyond the patient's control? Whether the barrier is transportation issues, financial concerns, or lack of understanding, the nurse can help advocate for alternative treatment options that can be both effective and accessible to the patient. The nurse sees beyond that patient's actions and understands that there are many barriers to what health care calls "compliance." In other words, the nurse treats the patients in the fullness of who they are.

We will say more about where nurses might go from here when we discuss the future of nursing in the third and final part of this book. But especially given already huge gaps in health-care systems around the developed West, and the growing gaps especially as our populations age, it is important to note that nurses have also been instrumental in filling in the gaps where the greatest needs exist. This is especially true for APRNs. In the early 1900s, nurse midwives traveled by horseback to reach underserved women and children.[29] By the 1960s, the first nurse practitioner training program was founded in order to meet the needs of a physician shortage throughout the nation.[30] And even today APRNs are traveling to rural or underserved communities and filling in the need for primary care for patients who would otherwise go without care.

With the aging population and changing health-care environment, there is now an even greater need for nurses to advocate for change to improve patient outcomes and access to care. Many health-care leaders and organizations have called on nurses to lead the change. The World Health Organization (WHO) designated 2020 as "The Year of the Nurse and Midwife."[31] Even the Institute of Medicine has called on nurses to become key players in health-care reform. In their report *The Future of Nursing*, they encouraged nurses to practice to the full extent of their education and training and be full partners, with physicians and other health professionals, in redesigning health care in the United States.[32] As the largest workforce in health care and the backbone of patient- and relationship-centered, whole-person care, nurses have not only the potential to lead health care into the future, but an obligation to patients to promote positive change in the care patients receive.

And Christian nurses should be especially confident in advocating for their more holistic understanding of the science, art, and spirituality present in their vocation—one that leads to offering patient-centered care in the fullness of who the patients are. Nurses are ready to lead the health-care professions into the future.

With that myth busted, let us turn to the final myth we will tackle in this first part of the book. Namely, the idea that faith and science—or faith and health care—"don't mix."

DISCUSSION QUESTIONS

1. This chapter discussed the role of the Christian nurse. As you think about your vocation, what is your theology or theology of nursing? What ultimate concerns and values guide your practice? How do

you understand the goals of nursing and how do they shape the care you provide?

2. One key role of being a nurse is being a patient advocate. What exactly does this mean? In what ways do/will you advocate for your patients?
3. To what extent does the broader culture of health care still value nurses as mere assistants? Are there changes that can be made to fully incorporate nursing as its own profession into the practice of health care?

3

FAITH, SCIENCE, AND HEALTH CARE

> Science can purify religion from error and superstition; religion can purify science from idolatry and false absolutes. Each can draw the other into a wider world, a world in which both can flourish.
>
> – *Pope John Paul II*

We can't tell you how many times people we meet, especially when they learn a bit about our backgrounds and beliefs, offer us some version of "religion and science don't mix" or "I'm in health care too and I keep it separate from my faith." The cultural impulse to make this kind of separation is powerful, especially in the consumerist West, but it comes from a third kind of myth that we mean to bust.

In some ways, the myth has already been busted. For we've already seen millions and millions of nurses today not only see absolutely no contradiction, no reason to separate their faith from their practice of health care, but instead actively embrace the connections between the two. For many of these folks, faith is the very reason they got into health care in the first place. We've also seen the good historical ground on which these contemporary nurses stand: nursing (at least in the West) comes out of a specifically Christian context, and the first nurses were also heavily invested in their Christian faith.

Nor are these connections limited to nursing. In a groundbreaking Grand Rounds presentation at the University of Michigan Medical school arguing that doctors should take spirituality seriously, Dr. Kristin Collier highlighted the very high percentage of US physicians—65.2 percent—who believe in God. In some ways, despite our culture's bias against religion and faith in medicine, this high number shouldn't surprise us. Collier also cites recent Pew poll data indicating that when asked "Do you believe in God?" about 80 percent answered yes; of those about 70 percent said they believed in God as described in the Bible and the rest in some other higher power or spiritual force. Of the 20 percent who answered no regarding belief in God, about half also nevertheless professed belief in some higher power or spiritual force. Only about 10 percent of respondents, then, did not believe in God or in any higher power or spiritual force. The 90 percent number for those who believe in God or some kind of spiritual being or force is high enough, but the data has also shown that people of color are significantly more religious than are whites. Collier highlighted Pew numbers which show that a whopping 75 percent of African Americans, for instance, say that religion is very important to them—with Hispanics at 59 percent and whites at 49 percent. Significant numbers for our racial justice moment.[1]

FROM WHERE DOES THIS MYTH COME?

Despite these facts, many nurses and nursing students still feel pressure to bracket off their Christian faith from their study of science and their practice of health care. In some ways, this pressure goes all the way back to the history and science many US Americans were taught in middle school and high school about the debates over evolution, and especially in what we were taught about the Galileo affair. In these classes, students are most often told that religion and science are not only two separate domains, but that their relationship should be thought of as adversarial. The image we are given is something like a zero-sum game which involves fighting for a kind of territory to explain the world around us. Whatever ground "one side" gains is ground "the other side" loses. In a health-care context, the debate is often set up between the side of rationality and good sense of science vs. the side of irrationality and superstition. When the terms of the conversation are established like this, it is not difficult to understand why a nurse or nursing student would be tempted to make a separation between their faith and their study and practice of science and health care.

The shift toward health care being a business has also contributed to the myths behind this divide. Hospitals are now places dominated by expensive technological intervention aimed at curing. Caring, so central to nursing, has taken a back seat to more profitable interventions. Many nurses express concern that nursing has continued to move farther away from the bedside while being substituted with a long list of procedures and tasks. In a related story, medicine often perceives that their authority comes exclusively from their technical training and use of the scientific method to diagnose and cure. Again, this training and level of expertise is important. But, the act of caring must also be infused into all acts of care in order for patients to receive the best possible care. And because health-care providers are paid to cure, not care, health care has become perplexed by the reality of death and totally geared toward avoiding or forestalling it. When death becomes imminent, it is then that "religion" takes over and "medicine" fades into the background.[2] Medicine, at least understood this way, is about only the biological flourishing of physical life. Goods which go beyond such a flat and one-dimensional understanding of what matters in health care fall outside the sphere of concern of those who currently get to decide what health care is for. Thus, health care becomes merely about using technical means for attending to the functioning of organic machines, while caring for people in the fullness of who they are (including their spiritual realities) is pushed to those outside of what we typically think of as the health-care professions—like the hospital chaplain or the patient's pastor.

A third significant reason science and medicine tend to keep separate from faith and spirituality is because of a perceived threat to their autonomy and freedom that some in the former group sense coming from some in the latter group. And this concern is not between different professions within health care, but about those who practice from a strictly science-based belief vs. those who believe in the importance of being guided by both science and religion. The former, who don't believe science and faith can mix, can feel threatened by those who do.

Where do religious traditions get off, they ask, telling scientists and health-care providers what to do in their research and medical practices? Don't they know their place? Professionals trained in these fields should be the ones to decide what is acceptable and what is not. The minute religious figures start pontificating about, say, whether it is acceptable to do gender reassignment surgery, or which kinds of abortions are permitted and which are not, it is clear that they have left the lane appropriate to their place in the culture. Don't bring the church into the clinic. Worship whatever god you like on your own time, but leave health-care providers alone to do what we know is best medically for patients and for advancing the progress of medicine.

We imagine a number of readers disagree with claims like these. And there is a good response to them. Such a response begins with getting the history of these matters right.

GETTING GALILEO WRONG

In at least in our experience, few people who work in health care know the religious history of their field as we've seen it explained in the previous two chapters. It would, therefore, be anything but surprising to discover that few know the actual history of the Galileo affair as well. Indeed, this may be the most misunderstood historical event in our culture at the moment. And given the dramatic effect that it has had on our cultural imagination—and particularly our culture's understanding of the relationship between science and faith—it is probably also fair to say it is our most significant historical misunderstanding as well.

Again, our current narrative goes something like this: Galileo was the data-driven scientist who bravely stood up to a superstitious religious institution, the Catholic Church, which didn't yet realize that it needed to stay in its lane and let scientists be in charge of science. Unfortunately, there was a time when superstitious institutions had power, and the Church used this power to imprison and torture Galileo and force him to recant his position that the earth moves around the sun and not the sun around the earth. But now we know better. We not only know that Galileo was justified in his claims—because he was backed up by rationality and evidence, not superstition—we also know that scientists must be given their autonomy and freedom apart from the claims of religious institutions and beliefs. When these two mix, it ends up limiting or even preventing the progress of science and extends faith beyond the limits of what it can properly access and address.

This narrative, while fundamentally mistaken, is not one hundred percent wrong. Though the Church never came close to torturing Galileo, its leaders did put him under house arrest and obviously did step outside the Church's proper lane by using temporal power to subject a scientist to legal accountability. Beyond that point, however, virtually every other part of the narrative most of us have been taught in school is mistaken.[3] Galileo was actually quite popular with many of the Church leaders of his day, and they were enthralled by his new theories. His basic claims about the relative motion of the earth and the sun, however, were not new. Nicholas Copernicus, who may well have been a priest or cleric of some kind (he was apparently a candidate to be cardinal at one point), came up with this idea well before Galileo and it was one of several competing theories among the scientists of the day. Everyone, including those who disagreed with him on the scientific merits, was totally fine with Galileo treating his theories as forming the basis for a serious and predictive, but unproven, hypothesis.

Given that they believed he had not proven his case, Church leaders resisted Galileo's demands that they change their interpretation of the Bible (especially at a time when Protestants were pushing Catholics to take the literal sense of Scripture more seriously), which appeared to claim that the sun moved around a stationary earth. These same Church leaders were very well aware of the scientific debates of the time and very often offered explicit financial and other support to Galileo and other scientists so they could do their work. Cardinal Robert Bellarmine, one of Galileo's most important conversation partners over the seventeen-year controversy, was so committed to the scientific evidence that he once claimed in a letter he wrote in April of 1615 that if Galileo proved his case scientifically, then the Church would be forced to change its interpretation of Scripture on the motion of heavenly bodies:

> I say that if there were a true demonstration that the sun is at the center of the world and the earth in the third heaven, and that the sun does not circle the earth but the earth circles the sun, then one would have to proceed with great care in explaining the Scriptures that appear contrary; and say rather that we do not understand them than that what is demonstrated is false. But I will not believe that there is such a demonstration, until it is shown me.[4]

Though this is not what we are generally taught in school, Galileo had indeed not proven his case.[5] He had even made several mistakes, like claiming that the ocean tides were a kind of sloshing in response to the movement of the earth rather than the effect of the moon's gravity—a view he described as childish.[6] He was also unable to account for the stellar parallax: the idea that, if the sun were stationary in relation to the earth, the stars would discernibly shift in our view every six months. Indeed, this objection was a primary reason many astronomers of Galileo's day (and for many centuries before) could not ultimately bring themselves to accept a heliocentric model.

Given these historical facts, the role that our culture typically ascribes to Galileo—one in which he, armed with his scientific theories, challenges the Church's mistaken understanding of Scripture—seems far less heroic and much more arrogant. Galileo should have also stayed in his lane, and first proven his own case, before he demanded that centuries of scriptural interpretation be overturned. The Church, maybe unsurprisingly given what we've already learned about its relationship to medicine, cared deeply about the scientific evidence and saw no contradiction between the goals of faith and the goals of science. Indeed, the history of science is filled with deeply religious people—from Copernicus to Newton to Leibniz to Mendel to Lemaître (and many thousands of others)—who believed that studying science was a window into learning about the Creator of the universe.

The almost certainly apocryphal saying attributed to Galileo—that the Church should stick to discussing "how to get to heaven, not how the heavens go"—nevertheless lingers. And the saying has some plausibility to it. Maybe it was OK to do in the past, but why should religious people and organizations dip their nose into complex matters of science and medicine today? Shouldn't the practice of contemporary medicine be a purely secular enterprise?

These are important questions. They also have important answers.

WHY PRACTICING SECULAR MEDICINE IS IMPOSSIBLE

Again, if the story being told is one in which medicine is about rational, procedural, careful, evidence-based practices—while religion is seen as dangerous superstition which can do little besides muck-up the process—it is understandable why someone might want to practice "secular" medicine. This is especially true if part of the mucking-up one has in mind involves a kind of censorship of medicine which impedes its ability to process in serving patients. The irreligious Canadian bioethicist Udo Schuklenk, for instance, argued in the prestigious *Journal of Medical Ethics* that would-be religious health-care providers should either check their faith at the door in the interests of "professionalism" or abandon the health-care professions altogether.[7] He also insists that, if religious health care-providers reject his point of view on this, they "prioritize their private beliefs, ultimately, over patient well-being."[8]

But here is where the problem comes in. There simply is no way for a health-care provider to act for a patient's good, for their "well-being," without *having a vision of the good in the first place.* We suppose it could be the very thin version of the good mentioned above: merely fixing and maintaining organic machinery. And if that's the view, then bringing up one's particular vision of the good may indeed seem strange or even off-putting. But we have already established in some detail that this a totally impoverished and one-dimensional view of what health-care providers do. They are far more than fixers and maintainers of organic machines. They care for people, often extremely vulnerable people, at some of the most significant moments of their lives. As we will discuss in some detail in Part II of the book, the massively important values at stake in these human interactions can produce very significant issues of ethics and morality.

These questions, and hundreds of others like them, can be answered only by appealing to fundamental values based on a particular vision of what is ultimately good and true. There is no secular "view from nowhere" in which we can distinguish between those who are doing this objectively and rationally (akin to using the scientific method for ethics) and those who are appealing to merely their own private opinion. Decisions about these matters can only be made on the basis of goods and values which transcend the immanent concerns on which secular Western medicine claims to be exclusively focused. It does no good to refer to "patient well-being" as if we can all agree on what that is in any particular circumstance—much less when there is white-hot disagreement in the culture about the particular goods and truths involved. Secular utilitarians, Muslim human rights activists, reproductive justice feminists, Catholic virtue ethicists, libertarian nationalists, Bible-focused evangelicals, atheistic anarchists, Jewish casuists—that is, *every single one of us*—must bring our own particular understandings of the good and true to bear on questions of bioethics. There is no way to avoid it.

And unless one wishes to simply single out religious visions of the good for special scrutiny (which at least seems a lot like bigotry) there is simply no way to practice "secular" medicine. If we are truly open-minded and tolerant as a (medical) culture in having an exchange of ideas about what is ultimately good and true, then we must welcome both religious and non-religious answers to these questions.

How all of this works in the real world may still seem a bit abstract. Let us focus on a particular historical example that may help us see this more clearly: how religious people with a certain vision of what is ultimately good about human beings clashed with the very different views on this topic offered by eugenic scientists and physicians.

THE EXAMPLE OF EUGENICS

Many are aware of the terrible Nazi eugenic practices in the era leading up to World War II. Fewer know that the ideology was particularly strong in the United States as well—and that some historians maintain that it was US eugenic ideology that inspired the Nazi version. The renowned Harvard biologist Charles Davenport, for instance, was an undisputed leader of the eugenics movement in the United States—and he generated a significant amount of scientific literature on what was thought to be the ill effects of bad decisions with regard to having children. Proceeding with the racist, classist, and ableist view that certain populations were "unfit" and ought not to bring more of their ilk into the world, eugenicists like Davenport gained popularity throughout the US and several other places around the world. He had significant connections to Nazi Germany and several eugenic activists there were influenced by his work. Here are three quotes from Davenport's eugenics creed:[9]

> I believe that I am the trustee of the germ plasm that I carry; that this has been passed on to me through thousands of generations before me; and that I betray the trust if (that germ plasm being good) I so act as to jeopardize it, with its excellent possibilities, or, from motives of personal convenience, to unduly limit offspring.
>
> I believe that, having made our choice in marriage carefully, we, the married pair, should seek to have 4 to 6 children in order that our carefully selected germ plasm shall be reproduced in adequate degree and that this preferred stock shall not be swamped by that less carefully selected.
>
> I believe in such a selection of immigrants as shall not tend to adulterate our national germ plasm with socially unfit traits.

Views like Davenport's found many sympathetic ears, especially among the privileged classes, and particularly at elite secular institutions, like Harvard.[10]

Nurses, as one might well imagine, were at the heart of many of the eugenic practices in the United States, the United Kingdom, Germany, and other places in the developed West during the first half of the twentieth century. Indeed, the shift we discussed in the previous chapter—the one in which nursing moved from having its own professional stature to nurses merely becoming assistants to doctors—was at least partially responsible for the complicity of many nurses in the medical practices of this era. The Christian vision of nursing provided by Moore and Nightingale, especially as discussed in chapter 1, imagines a profession that would never countenance blind obedience to physicians, but instead proposes an interaction of two professionals in which both sets of concerns were respected. By the time the era of eugenics rolled around, however, that model had been replaced by one in which nurses were "obliged to act according to the policies and directives issued by authorities in all fields of health care."[11] This secular and subservient context was quite different from the one assumed by Moore and Nightingale, and it led not a few nurses to dutifully, yet complicitly, participate in all sorts of terrible eugenic practices—including hundreds of thousands of forced sterilizations.[12] It is important to point out that there were many nurses who would not participate because of their faith, however, and they had to pay the cost for their "disobedience."

Eugenic practices did receive significant resistance, however, especially from Catholics and more traditional Protestant Christians.[13] Just as the practice was gaining widespread popular, scientific, and legal momentum in the developed West, Pope Pius XII released a counter-cultural encyclical calling eugenics a "grave crime" and "pernicious practice."[14] In the United States, Monsignor John A. Ryan, a scholar and activist on Catholic social teaching, artfully took the fight to the American Eugenics Society with special focus from the anti-consumerism perspective of his Christian faith.[15]

There was even significant Christian resistance within Nazi Germany itself as the terrible logic of eugenics unfolded with the murderous policies of the Third Reich. While many nurses abandoned their professional duties to care for the most vulnerable by implementing the Nazi euthanasia program, a significant number of nurses refused to participate. Particularly inspired by the active resistance to the Nazi euthanasia program by Bishop Clemens August van Galen, public reaction and even civil unrest became such a threat to the Nazi hold on power that it undermined the whole program. According to the historian Richard J. Evans, "[n]urses and orderlies, especially in Catholic institutions for the sick and the disabled," were able "seriously to obstruct the process of registration."[16] Sister Anna Bertha Königsegg, a member of the Congregation of the Sisters of Mercy of St. Vincent de Paul, was one of the most important leaders of the resistance against the "T4" euthanasia program and forced sterilizations of the disabled.[17] She was arrested by the Gestapo, and later the whole Congregation had their property confiscated throughout the Reich, but the general resistance they embodied was growing and that was apparently enough for Hitler to stop his euthanasia program, at least for disabled adults.

A CHRISTIAN VISION OF BIOETHICS

The vision of the good operative in the Christian resistance to medical eugenics came from—to use Professor Schuklenk's language—prioritizing their private beliefs. These private beliefs were at odds with those who held power in the local culture, but they were nevertheless an essential part of what now all see as an essential good: resisting Nazi medicine. Questions of ethics and values are necessary for discussing the very essence of health care itself. By its very nature, asking the question "What does good health care look like?" transcends the practice of health care. One needs to step out of the practice to ask about what health care is for.

And here is where traditions of thought that make claims about what is ultimately good and true step in to answer such questions. Not only is it wrong to keep such traditions out of the discussion of medicine and health care, *we can't even claim to know what medicine and health care are for in the first place* without appealing to them. And the oldest tradition we have in this space, the one that goes back to the very beginnings of how the developed West began to think about health care and nursing, is the Christian tradition.

Perhaps it is more accurate to say Christian traditions. We, ourselves, represent two different strains of Christianity: Alisha is an evangelical Protestant and Charlie is a Roman Catholic. And though we don't agree on everything, in the chapter that follows, we articulate a common Christian theological vision that will establish the ethical principles we will use throughout the rest of the book to show what a bioethics for Christian nurses looks like.

Let us keep the central lesson of this chapter in mind as we move forward through the second part of the book. Not only is it a bad idea to keep these kinds of discussions out of health care and nursing, we can't even talk about what nursing or health care is in the first place without addressing what this second part of the book tackles.

DISCUSSION QUESTIONS

1. This chapter presents the argument that practicing secular medicine is impossible. Do you agree with the argument made? Why or why not?
2. You just read about eugenic practices performed by health-care providers less than a century ago. Today the thought of what occurred in

the United States and in Nazi Germany is hard for anyone to fathom, but are eugenic practices and impulses still around today? What practices in our current health-care system do you think others will look back on years from now and find difficult to fathom?

3. This chapter presents the argument that there is simply no way for a health-care provider to act for a patient's good without having a vision of the good in the first place. In a health-care setting, your vision of the good as a health-care provider may conflict with the vision of the good of the patient. How do you view these two visions of the good—that is, is one more important than the other?

4

A CHRISTIAN VISION FOR NURSING BIOETHICS

> Where there is no vision, the people perish.
>
> – *Proverbs 29:18 (KJV)*

The Christian vision we present in this chapter did not emerge from nowhere. It is grounded in the Scripture and Tradition of the Catholic Church, both of which are God-inspired works of ancient holy people who have gone before us. It is God's vision that has shaped us, not the other way around (as happens very often in a culture focused almost exclusively on individual expression of the autonomous will). We both had very different visions of what was ultimately true and good before the vision presented in this chapter compelled us to think and see differently. God's grace has changed our hearts and continues to sustain us even in the midst of a culture that is often hostile toward the vision we are about to present. We have not demanded that Scripture and Tradition change because of what we desired to see; instead, God's grace has transformed us so that we now see through gospel-tinted glasses.

There is a second sense in which this chapter does not spring out of nowhere. The three preceding chapters have already described this vision in substantial ways. For example, we have encountered the central idea that a Christian looks at everything through the life and teachings of Jesus Christ—with one obvious example being Christianity having such a focus on health and healing because this was such a priority for Jesus Himself. (Remarkably, nearly a third of the Gospel stories involve narratives related to healing.) In addition, by encountering Christian communities like the Sisters of Mercy and Samaritan's Purse, we have seen that Christ's commands to love in particular ways include putting God first and recognizing that everything rests on God. But we saw that it also means loving one's neighbor in ways that are connected to loving for oneself. We have also seen these communities live out Christ's great teaching that authentic power comes from service to others. Christian power dynamics work in a very different way from what the world tells us. Indeed, it turns the conventional wisdom of the world on its head: You want to be first? Put others before you. You want power? Embrace your weakness. You want glory? Embrace humility and even humiliation. Any authentic power we have comes from putting the love of the marginalized ahead of our own personal interests.

We also learn from the example of Florence Nightingale that one's calling to be a nurse is part of a broader calling from God, who invites us to our life's vocation. To the extent that we achieve any power through our service (as Nightingale herself did) she reminds us that we are unworthy of it and that the "highest expression" of faithfulness to God's call is the cross—the ultimate example of dying to self for others. Furthermore, she reminds us that loving others in a Christian context means serving them in the fullness of who they are. God created us, body and soul, in His divine image. Both are essential parts of who we are. Furthermore, God's spiritual reality is intimately intertwined with our own. Nightingale's service demonstrates that a human life is as intimate a work of art as we can imagine, for the artist, God Himself, had made his home in we humans, who are temples of the Holy Spirit. Nurses, if they are going to serve people in their full reality, are not just skilled technicians working with other skilled technicians trying to fix or maintain an organic machine. On the contrary, Nightingale reminds us that nursing is an art. Her approach to health care here, again, imitates the example of Christ whose own example of service to the sick focused both on physical and spiritual healing together.

A Christ follower's love needs to be impartial in the sense of not blinded by confirmation bias and self-interest, as we saw in the values of the Sisters of Mercy. But the sisters also demonstrate that it is *not* impartial in another sense: for our love must give priority to people in whom Christ dwells in a particular way. That is, we must have a special priority for "least ones," those who are pushed to the margins of the culture. We see in Matthew 25 how our service to the hungry, thirsty, stranger, naked, and imprisoned is not only service to Christ himself, but representative of the kind of life that separates the sheep from the goats—from those who will have union with God forever and ever and those who will not. How this kind of marginalization manifests itself will often vary from culture to culture, especially given that what it can mean to be the "least" among us is dependent on many different social factors. In one culture, for instance, a prenatal child or an immigrant might be welcomed as a living symbol of the future and vitality of the society, while in another they might be thought of as burdensome and foreign "parasites" who should not be welcomed. The imitation of Christ, however, means critiquing those who are close to political, institutional, and other kinds of power in whatever social context they push the least among us to the margins and refuse to honor the special way in which they bear the face of the Lord.

BUT WHY SHOULD WE IMITATE CHRIST, AGAIN?

Why should anyone imitate an ancient Jewish itinerant preacher and healer from the rural area of Nazareth? Why would nurses like Mary Clare Moore and Florence Nightingale devote their entire lives in such profound ways to this particular person? To begin to answer these questions, it is important to do some thinking about what religious beliefs are in the first place. As mentioned in the previous chapter, there is no "view from nowhere" when it comes to thinking about what is involved in good health care and nursing. Doing a deep exploration of this requires a particular vision of the good in the first place. Such a vision comes out of what some thinkers call "first principles," those foundational and irreducible values which point our lives in particular directions and along particular trajectories toward particular goals or ends. Human beings are the kind of creatures who, when healthy and mature, make sense and meaning out of the world around them—particularly when they choose to orient their lives toward their ultimate concern or concerns. This is simply part of the human condition and is true both of those who are explicitly religious and those who are not. The question is not whether one will serve a god or gods (lower-case "g" is intentional), but which god or gods they choose to serve. It is here, in these kinds of life decisions, that human beings reveal what they believe to be of ultimate value or concern. For some it is consumerism. Others put their country first. For still others it is social acceptance and validation, especially via social media. And for a good chunk of people there are multiple irreducible sources of ultimate concern. Many are functional polytheists.[1]

For Christians (along with Jews and Muslims), however, there can be only one ultimate concern: God. This is what it means to be a monotheist. All other candidates for ultimate concern, those that are rivals for the one true God, are ruled out by the First Commandment of the Decalogue of the Hebrew Bible or (for Christians) the Old Testament. Idolatry in today's context is no longer a worry about a bowing down before golden idols or offering a pinch of incense to Jupiter or Caesar. No, today's Christians speak out against the worship of gods like money, sex, and nationalism. This view does not imply that there are no other values or other good things in the world. There most certainly are: in fact, God created them good. But there is only one *ultimate* good. The source of all other goods and that to which all other goods must be directed: God.

And Christians know from Scripture, tradition, and our own experience of this God that he has a particular nature: diversity in unity, plurality in singularity, one being whose very essence is to be in relationship. Three persons—the Father, Son, and Holy Spirit—in one divine being. This triune God sent his only Son, the Divine Word, to be incarnated in the flesh of a human being, Jesus the Christ: the name which is above all other names. This Jesus is the visible image of the invisible God. And here we have the answer to the question, "Why should anyone imitate an ancient Jewish itinerant preacher and healer from Nazareth?" The answer is because this person was and remains God himself, who came to show us—through an intimate relationship with him—that we can live as God wants us to live.

That this can happen at all is a great mystery: for how can the infinite and divine interact with the finite and human? The best Christians can do in answering this massive question (beyond invoking our own spiritual experiences and those of our religious ancestors of Jesus as God) is to point to the biblical example of this convergence of the human and the divine happening in the person of an ancient Jewish itinerant preacher and healer from Nazareth. He who received power through submissive obedience to his divine Father, with whom he claimed an astonishing kind of unity and familiarity. He who gained glory by living among and serving the lowly and wretched of his day. Whose resurrection defeated death only after his refusal to resist a humiliating and terrible crucifixion at the hands of an empire that those who took a more traditional view of power mistakenly thought he would overthrow. This is the person Christians have come to know, through faith, who has revealed God most clearly and directly to us.

CHRIST AS REDEEMER AND REVEALER OF WHAT IT MEANS TO BE HUMAN

The human and divine are connected in such a powerful way in the incarnation of God in the person of Jesus that it gives new meaning to the first chapter of Genesis saying that God made human beings in God's holy and divine image. That image was strained and even disfigured due to our sin, but through Christ's sacrifice and resurrection our human nature (and even in certain parts of Scripture and tradition, our literal flesh—*sarx*—is emphasized) has been redeemed as holy. The person of Jesus Christ not only reveals most clearly what God is like, he reveals the authentic nature of human beings as well. And though we are clearly spirit in that we have souls, we are also essentially embodied creatures. The Bible is at great pains to emphasize Jesus's body, especially after the resurrection. It was a glorified body, to be sure, but the Gospels deliberately emphasize that the body of Jesus after the resurrection ate food (something that ghosts or spirits alone do not do) and that Thomas was invited to touch the wounds that still remained in Jesus's hands and side from the crucifixion. This is one important reason why the early church would specifically affirm "the resurrection of the body" for human beings in the Nicene Creed.

So, the particular nature of human beings is to be, in the very essence of who we are, body and spirit at the same time. To focus on one to the exclusion of the other misses something essential about who and what we are. And as we have seen and will see many times throughout this book, any focus on health care of a human being in the fullness of who they are will take into account both aspects of our human nature. We have this nature as individuals—having been created in the image and likeness of God and have been personally redeemed by Christ—and this gives each one of us inherent dignity that cannot be collapsed into a utilitarian-like calculation about maximizing the greatest good for the greatest number. Again, the dignity of the most vulnerable human beings deserves our special attention. But having been created in the image and likeness of a *triune* God, a God whose very essence is to be in relationship, we know that we are not created as isolated individuals. On the contrary, the incarnation has made us all brothers and sisters in Christ, and this means that we are deeply and profoundly related to all other human beings. What makes us different from each other may be interesting and significant, but in the essence of who we are, we are all equal and united in our common humanity. As Saint Paul reminds us: there is neither Jew nor Gentile, neither slave nor free, nor is there male and female. We are all one in Christ Jesus.

This means that Christians must be wary of the American culture's tendency toward individualism. Too often we see our relationships with others as a burden to our individual freedom and autonomy. But this image of the radically autonomous free agent, able to exert our individual will without the limitations of our creaturely finitude and obligations to others, is not consistent with a Christian vision of the inherent relationality between human beings. On the contrary, if we start by acknowledging the fact that we have been created as human animals, members of the species *Homo sapiens*, we cannot help but also acknowledge the givenness of the limitations of our embodied natures. We cannot simply reshape who and what we are. We are not radically free to choose to become or do whatever we wish. Not only do we have the givenness of our created human natures, but also the givenness of the relationships and the obligations which come with them. The duty to honor our mother, for example, is simply a given in our lives—the situation into which we have been dropped.

The givenness of our created nature as a human organism (though an organism that is a temple of God's Holy Spirit) becomes important, even essential, to several ideas at the heart of important bioethical issues we will discuss later in this book. For instance, as finite beings who are not our own creators, we do not in any sense "own" our bodies or our lives. They belong to our Creator and must be ultimately directed toward him. In addition, a focus on science (which is something Christians should embrace as revealing much about the being who created us) reveals our beginning and end of our lives on this earth as human organisms. What we now know about prenatal development of the human being is quite consistent with Scripture's claim that God formed and knit us together in our mother's womb, for the prenatal human being is no less a member of the species *Homo sapiens* than is any reader of this book. Likewise, our lives as human beings do not end when a single organ (even the brain) suffers a catastrophic injury or disease. We die when our human bodies die, not when we lose certain capacities like rationality, self-awareness, memory, language, or the like. Again, in Christ we are all equal, all brothers and sisters, apart from contingent properties. All living human beings share the same human nature. This is what makes us equal.

So theologically speaking, what can we say about human beings from what we've discussed in the paragraphs above? Let us highlight some key points for emphasis:

- Human beings are embodied, finite creatures, made in the image and likeness of their Creator, a Creator who has made his home in us in a special way as temples of the Holy Spirit.
- We have defiled and disfigured that image and likeness, but God sent His only Son—Jesus, the Christ—to save us and redeem us. Human beings (and even human *sarx* itself) have been redeemed and made holy through the incarnation of God in the human person of Jesus.
- All human beings are equal, not based on this or that trait, but rather as fellow living human beings with a shared dignified nature—from the beginning of the human organism to the death of that organism.
- This shared human nature is given to us by our Creator. In this sense we do not own our bodies or our lives, but owe them to God and must point our life's trajectory back toward our Creator.

- Our Creator is a Trinity—three persons (Father, Son, and Holy Spirit) in one being—and is essentially relational. Human beings reflect God's inherent relationality in our own natures. We are individuals, yes, and have inherent dignity from being created and loved by God as individuals. But we are also inherently relational, and our flourishing as the kinds of creatures we are cannot be expressed apart from relationships with (and unchosen obligations toward) others.

That final bullet point deserves more attention. Through a personal relationship with him, we learn about God and about what and who authentic human beings are. But we also learn about the kind of life our divine creator is calling human beings to; we learn about what kinds of relationships we should have with others. And it is to this essential topic we now turn.

WHAT KIND OF RELATIONSHIPS SHOULD WE HAVE WITH OTHERS?

The kind of life to which God is calling us is a central concern for current and future nurses, for Christian ethics, and for current and future nurses interested in Christian bioethics. Based on what has been said above, it should surprise no one that Christians look to both imitate and obey Christ in this regard. Christ, the visible image of the invisible God, reveals a God who is love. Again, relationship is the essence of who God is. Not just any kind of relationship is revealed: it is a relationship based on love that is both impartial in some ways (Jesus poignantly prays in the Garden of Gethsemane that the Father's will be done, not his own) and partial in others (Jesus's service is to the least ones). God calls us to engage in similarly loving relationships as well. One way he does this is by his example: indeed, His command to "love one another, as I have loved you" is clear in this regard (John 13:34 KJV). His other commands, including what he says are the two greatest commandments, also put love at the center of the Christian life.

First, we are commanded to love God with everything that we are: our whole heart, soul, mind, and strength. And the second-greatest commandment, which Christ says is like the first, is to love our neighbor as ourselves (Matt. 22:37–29; Mark 12:29–31).

Interestingly, in Luke's Gospel (the author of which was for many centuries thought to be a professional provider of health care, though this is now disputed), the discussion of these two commandments is followed by Jesus offering the parable of the Good Samaritan as a way of helping to explain what neighbor love looks like. And it should come as no surprise to Christians interested in nursing, many of whom may have been deeply influenced by the Good Samaritan, that this parable has become foundational for how many Christians have thought about Christ-centered love via health care.[2] After all, Jesus commands us to "go and do likewise" after telling this story in Luke 10.

But what is it that we should do? The first and most obvious practice revealed by the parable is going out of our way to aid those who are most in need. The "better classes" of people in the story crossed to the other side of the road precisely to avoid having to confront the man who was assaulted by robbers, but the Good Samaritan refused to alter his path and allowed himself to be confronted with the injured man's great need. This reminds Charlie of a story he heard from a certified nursing assistant (CNA) working on the dementia floor of a nursing home during the COVID-19 pandemic. While she and other nursing staff were terribly overworked and refused to quit in the face of terrible burdens, some of the physicians she worked with were most often nowhere to be found. Indeed, even some of the podiatrists refused to show up on their floor, with the result that her patients very often had significant and even disgusting foot ailments due to lack of care. Meanwhile, like the Good Samaritan, the nurses and CNAs drew near to the vulnerable they encountered and took responsibility for their care.

The Good Samaritan, who is "moved with compassion" (Luke 10:33), has a heart which helps him see those in need—to see the profound, inestimable value of human life, even when it is injured, sick, fragile, or weak. This is very different from the kind of heart produced by what Pope Francis calls a throwaway culture: a heart that has been blinded to the needs of those who are pushed to the margins. Especially given that many of us are products of such a culture and often driven by an idolatrous consumerism, many of us have needed the grace of God to change our sinful hearts from the kinds that are too busy, too important, or too self-absorbed to genuinely encounter and take responsibility for someone who needs us. Indeed, the Good Samaritan not only tends to the wounds of the vulnerable person, he stops his journey, puts the injured man on his own animal, and purchases a room in which he can care for him.

This puts on display another calling that Christians have to the sick and injured: accompaniment. Here we are reminded of Christ's own sufferings in the Garden of Gethsemane, before which he asked his disciples to stay up and watch him while he prayed. Christian nurses are called not only to bind up the wounds of patients, but in the spirit of mercy to be physically close to patients in their illness, keeping vigil so they do not suffer loneliness in their final days and hours. This kind of care—at which nurses are so skilled—has physical benefits for patients to be sure, but it also has spiritual ones. It respects the fullness of the dignity of the human being who, again, was created to be in relationships with others. Indeed, the particular relationship between patient and nurse means that the latter must be willing to suffer with the former. Indeed, the word "compassion" literally means to "suffer with."

This is especially important—for both patient and family alike—when little can be done other than palliative care. Such care is not an abandonment of the person, but rather a powerful example of accompanying a patient in the final days of their existence. Christians who are aware of our own finitude and firm in the gift of hope given by the Holy Spirit of a more perfect union with God, do not avoid death at all costs. We rather come to accept it as a natural part of our creaturely life. Indeed, Saint Francis of Assisi came to speak of "Sister Death" toward the end of his life, especially as he more fully accepted what death and resurrection mean for all of us.[3] Health-care providers accepting the reality of death, however, must never abandon or discard a dying patient. On the contrary, this is perhaps the most important time to be lovingly present to everyone involved, for a culture that denies death as much as ours does can make facing the truth of how this life ends that much more difficult. Spiritually-grounded nurses, guided by the gift of hope in the supernatural horizon of the lives of human beings, can care for the whole person even when medicine exhausted what it can do.

NONVIOLENT HEALTH CARE

A good death, then, is one in which the supernatural hope in a horizon beyond the one in this life is firmly in view. It is supported by those who, while emphasizing this hope, refuse to abandon the dignity and present needs of the still living patient, especially via palliative and spiritual care. Friends, family, and other caregivers keep vigil, accompanying the patient on their final journey of this life, accepting death as part of what it means to be finite. But accepting death is not the same as seeking it out. Jesus accepted the will of the Father that he was to die on the cross, but he did not aim at his own death. On the contrary, during his agony in the Garden of Gethsemane Jesus prayed to the Father that the cup would pass from him. In being obedient even unto death, however, Jesus modeled what it means to live out truth that our lives ultimately belong to our Creator, not to us. We don't get to decide when we come into this world, and we don't get to decide when we leave it. And we certainly don't get to decide that for someone else. God himself is the Lord of life and of death. We are not.

This is one important reason for us to heed Christ's example and call to nonviolence. The commandment making killing inadmissible applies to the provider of health care in a particularly dramatic way. Genuine compassion—again, a willingness to "suffer with"—is not compatible with the violent snuffing out of life that is so characteristic of today's throwaway culture. Too often we speak of a burden on the patient as our reason to want them to "die with dignity" or "spare them suffering"—when in fact the burden is on us. *We* don't want to burden *ourselves* with what the compassionate care of the sick and dying requires. Indeed, fear of being such a burden on others is what drives many of those vulnerable people who request assisted suicide today. Instead of lazily slouching toward a culture which violently discards those who are sick, we should move toward nonviolent practices of accompaniment of those making their final journey of this life.

Authentic compassion and love for someone is, simply put, incompatible with killing them. Especially when it comes to heath care. The early church took Jesus Christ's call to nonviolence so seriously that they forbade Christians from joining the Roman army, claiming they were forbidden to shed blood.[4] Via the Didache, one of the earliest documents we have from the Christian church, we learn that they contrasted "the way of life" with "the way of death" in ways that forbade both abortion and infanticide, which were thought to be morally similar acts. Whether we are talking about the beginning of life, the very end of life, or anywhere in between, killing is never caring and can therefore never be a part of authentic health care.

Though it is under near constant assault by a secular medical culture (which has largely rejected its Christian roots), at the time this book goes to press the code of medical ethics from the American Medical Association still rejects assisted suicide as "fundamentally incompatible" with the role of the health-care provider.[5] Providers must focus on the goodness of the lives of human beings under their care, especially when they are in an incredibly vulnerable state, and demonstrate our willingness to stand firm with them during their final days and hours. Given what has just been said, it may not be surprising to learn that cultural slouches toward assisted suicide have deleterious effects on palliative and end-of-life care.[6] When Charlie's service-learning students in bioethics served at Calvary Hospice Center in the Bronx, they learned firsthand that no patient who was welcomed and valued by that extraordinary institution ever requested assisted suicide. The compassion and love they felt from the staff helped patients to see that their own lives were still worthy, even when they first arrived feeling profound anguish and despair. And Alisha witnessed this many times throughout her years working in the hospital. She would argue that to be with someone in their final hours, to hold their hand and tell them they are not alone, and to comfort them through prayer—it is something that no words can describe. It is one of the most intimate and extraordinary experiences between two humans. To be able to give someone peace as they make the journey out of this world, into the next, is one of the most powerful gifts we can give to another human being.

ARRIVING AT SEVEN KEY BIOETHICAL PRINCIPLES

There are central truths the Bible teaches that act as a moral compass when navigating the difficult (bio)ethical waters we are about to navigate. Some may argue that Scripture is unable to guide current ethical situations related to medicine since medicine (and especially medical technology) has developed and advanced since the time it was written. We appreciate this concern and acknowledge that modern technology has been the catalyst for many medical dilemmas found in health care today.[7] However, what is also true is that while the Bible may not mention specific ethical problems, ethical *concepts* can be derived from principles taught in Scripture.[8] In fact, we find this truth underscored in 2 Timothy 3:16–17: "All Scripture is God-breathed and is useful for teaching . . . so that the servant of God may be thoroughly equipped for every good work." Indeed, if there is an

Author above all authors of the Bible, then one should be able to derive moral guidance from the Bible at some deep level.[9] Furthermore, many Christians believe that God continues to speak to us through tradition of the church and through the people of God today, to help guide us when genuinely new ideas come about.

As mentioned in the introduction to this book, we want to apply our Christian bioethical vision to the real world of health care. The whole of the preceding Christian vision will be operative in the next seven chapters, but each chapter will have a particular focus on one of the following seven key principles distilled from this vision:

1. Human beings have equal dignity and value from having been made in the image and likeness of God.
2. Human beings are living bodies (as well as spirits), and therefore begin our existence as human organisms after fertilization and end our existence when that human organism dies.
3. We must accept death when it comes without ever violently aiming at it.
4. All human beings, especially those who bear the Face of Christ in a special way as the least among us, are equal before God regardless of human-created distinctions.
5. We must put aside our selfish interests as understood by the world in favor of a "the last shall be first" love which, turning conventional wisdom on its head, puts a direct focus on those the surrounding culture has marginalized.
6. Human beings can only be fully ourselves in relationships with others, especially our families and those with whom we have genuine, embodied relationships.
7. We must love God with all our heart, all our soul, all our mind, and all our strength.

In each of the following seven chapters, though we will explore several different contexts in which nurses will put the above principles into action, we will focus in particular on one case study we believe illustrates the principle being emphasized in that chapter in a powerful or revealing way.

One final note: It is by now abundantly clear why we said at the beginning that this book is written primarily for Christian nurses. But while we see each principle through a Christian lens, it should also be said that versions of many of these principles are often held dear by non-Christians and even those with no faith at all when encountering a difficult ethical situation. Thus, much of the analysis of the cases which follow in the next several chapters can be the basis for productive discussion between Christian and non-Christian nurses.

But let us turn now to a discussion of our first principle: namely, that human beings have dignity and value from having been made in the image and likeness of God.

DISCUSSION QUESTIONS

1. This chapter focuses on the person of Jesus Christ and how he reveals the authentic nature of human beings, especially our embodied nature. How is your view of the human body (especially as it pertains to the vocation of nursing) influenced by your Christian faith?
2. Jesus is often called the Great Physician and has attributes that would be of great benefit for health-care providers to adopt. One of these attributes is discussed in this chapter: his practice of nonviolence. What other attributes of Christ are or will be particularly relevant to your work as a Christian nurse?
3. This chapter introduces seven key principles to guide Christian nursing practice. Are there certain principles that you feel are most important? Which principle(s) do you feel are difficult to practice given the current health-care environment?

PART TWO

Christian Nursing Bioethics in Action

5

MADE EQUAL IN THE DIVINE IMAGE

> If we have no peace, it is because we have forgotten that we belong to each other.
>
> – *Saint Teresa of Calcutta*

The first of the seven principles with which we concluded the previous chapter, and our guiding light for this chapter, is that human beings have dignity and value from having been made equal in the image and likeness of God. Our role as Christians is to fully understand and appreciate the uniqueness and beauty of each person, especially if the world does not recognize those characteristics. In fact, God calls us to run toward those whom the world tends to turn away from:

> Then Jesus said to his host, "When you give a luncheon or dinner, do not invite your friends, your brothers or sisters, your relatives, or your rich neighbors; if you do, they may invite you back and so you will be repaid. But when you give a banquet, invite the poor, the crippled, the lame, the blind, and you will be blessed. Although they cannot repay you, you will be repaid at the resurrection of the righteous." (Luke 14:12–14 NIV)

This vision is to be contrasted with other visions of dignity and worth in our culture, which tends to focus on the worth of certain traits or characteristics. Human beings on this view are valuable, not because they all bear the same image and likeness of God in the very nature of who they are, but only if they have some kind of morally relevant ability: rationality, self-awareness, autonomy, intelligence, productivity, and the like. Christianity utterly rejects this ableist vision of value in favor of one that affirms fundamental human dignity and essential human equality regardless of these accidental characteristics.

Let us now dive deeper into what this means for health care and the role Christian nurses play as it relates to this principle.

HUMAN WORTH AND DIGNITY IN HEALTH CARE

History books are filled with examples of atrocities based on viewing certain groups of people as worthless; and more often than we may like to admit, these atrocities take place in the context of health care. We have already focused on how the Nazi regime murdered and euthanized millions of people during World War II based on the belief that people of certain races, religions, and disabilities were subhuman. How this type of brutality could have occurred bewilders us today, yet we are talking about something that happened less than a century ago. In order to understand how such crime against humanity could take place, it is essential to recognize that it did not begin overnight—but rather through small changes in beliefs and influence. At the beginning of this chapter on human dignity, it is important to understand how these small changes began.

Dr. Leo Alexander was an American physician and key medical advisor during the Nuremberg trials (trials to bring justice for crimes the Nazi war criminals committed). He wrote about the atrocities in a landmark article in *The New England Journal of Medicine* in 1949. He discussed the complicity of health-care providers during the Nazi regime. One of his statements, which is perhaps the most relevant to this discussion on human worth, examines the beginning of the crimes:[1]

> Whatever proportions these crimes finally assumed, it became evident to all who investigated that they had started from small beginnings. The beginnings at first were merely a subtle shift in emphasis in the basic attitude of the physicians. It started with the acceptance of the attitude, basic in the euthanasia movement, that there is such a thing as life not worthy to be lived.
>
> This attitude in its early stages concerned itself merely with the severely and chronically sick. Gradually, the sphere of those to be included in this category was enlarged to encompass the socially unproductive, the ideologically unwanted, the racially unwanted, and, finally, all non-Germans.[2]

Dr. Alexander highlights a key point: the change in practice started with making exceptions to justify morally-conflicting practices. How many practices have crept into medical care that have slowly become acceptable, or even common practice, that go against our duty to protect and do no harm? They are often similarly camouflaged as a just and moral act for a greater cause.

During the Nuremberg Trials folks started to speak about something called the "Eichmann Effect"—the willingness to commit offenses one would not normally commit when one sees themselves as merely an instrument of some higher authority. Could something similar be affecting health-care providers who, while working to protect society, subtly make it easier to eliminate those who are a "burden" to it? In order to get to this accepted practice, a society must dehumanize the target population, since most societies view killing a human being with inherent dignity as morally wrong. So, those populations must first be demoted from humans to nonhumans, or subhumans.[3]

This is not merely a concern of the past. There are many different areas in health care today in which this concern surfaces. Human worth is the underlying factor when it comes to abortion and physician-assisted suicide, but also in situations like resource allocation, health-care discrimination, and denial of care. As we've said many times throughout this book, having values and a vision of the good is an essential part of what it means to practice health care.

HUMAN DIGNITY AND EQUALITY IN NURSING CARE

Nurses across all areas in health care—obstetrics, pediatrics, intensive care, medical-surgical, school-based, elder care, and more—have faced situations in which they are asked to proceed either as if all human lives are fundamentally equal or as if some lives matter more than others because of valuable traits or abilities they do or do not have. Nearly every nurse, for instance, has dealt with issues of being short-staffed—an issue that is becoming a growing national problem and one which presents major concerns related to human dignity and equality for hospital and other clinical administrators. There is an emerging body of literature that address what is termed "care left undone," and this reality is placed on nurses due to limited time and resources.[4] One group reports, "In the midst of multiple demands and inadequate resources, what choices do nurses make to provide the best care possible? There are times when they find it impossible to fulfil all nursing care requirements or choose not to complete all aspects of care for a variety of reasons. In these circumstances, nurses may abbreviate the care, may delay the care, or may simply omit the care."[5]

In these situations, nurses are forced to prioritize where they will focus their time and energy. Do they choose to allocate time to patients with the "best prognosis"? And is this about the recovering of the health of their bodies or is it about having a certain quality of life? What about disabled patients who require the most hands-on care? And what about, as we will discuss in greater detail in the chapter on nursing after the pandemic, the reasoning behind decisions to ration scarce supplies, equipment, and medication? This has become an increasing problem due to a growing population, higher life expectancy, higher cost of treatments, and a greater number of treatment options, among other reasons.[6]

There is no agreed-upon rule as to how to ration resources and staff when either is limited. The burden of making this decision has often been placed on the individual nurse in ways that are linked to moral distress.[7] But, the truth is that resources are limited, even for the wealthiest nations in the world.[8] We cannot assume that we can offer every patient every resource available, and difficult choices must be made on a daily basis. By focusing resources to one group, it inevitably decreases them for another. As a society, and as a health-care system, do we allocate more funding to preventive measures or cures? Do we put more funding toward fighting diseases that affect the young or the elderly, who typically have more comorbidities?[9] Or do we allocate resources evenly between each category? To say that these questions are difficult to answer is an understatement, but we must acknowledge that human dignity and equality are most under threat when there is a lack of resources. A Christian nurse, resisting the culture impulse to have some lives matter more than others, must always share the same starting point: the lives of all human beings matter the same regardless of their particular traits. It is their common natures—even if they are imperfectly expressed due to immaturity, injury, disease, age—that each reflect the image and likeness of God and therefore make them equal in dignity.

Especially if they are in a secular context, many nursing students and practicing nurses are likely to be confronted with the concept of "quality of life." And in one sense, Christian nurses ought to be very concerned with improving the quality of life of their patients. Easing their pain, making it easier for them to recover, helping instill practices that will lead to better long-term outcomes. But in a secular context, one's quality of life often has to do with abilities they may have that American consumer culture considers valuable. Quality of life is measured by whether patients are "productive members of society." When discussing disabilities, there is an implicit judgment that a disabled life is "less than" that of someone who is differently abled. But the act of caring for someone who is unable to care for themselves often causes more of a transformation of the caretakers than the patients themselves. One passage found in the Gospel of John even describes care and healing for the sick and disabled as revealing God's work: "As he went along, he saw a man blind from birth. His disciples asked him, 'Rabbi, who sinned, this man or his parents, that he was born blind?' 'Neither this man nor his parents sinned,' said Jesus, 'but this happened so that the works of God might be displayed in him'" (John 9:1–3).

We see this with a mother who cares for her infant. An infant, by nature, is incapable of taking care of himself. However, with each act of care—feeding, dressing, soothing—the mother's heart grows closer to her child and a love develops between the two. The mother does not choose to care for her child based on what she will get in return. She cares for her child out of love and dedication. The kind of care offered by nurses—to each and every human person as a bearer of God's image and likeness (and regardless of their traits)—can be similarly life-giving and displaying of the works of God.

Also like parents, nurses who care for children often have multiple ethical concerns. Children, by nature, require special and careful considerations because they often rely on someone else to protect them and to be their voice, whether it is an unborn child, a newborn, a child with a disability, or a child with incapacitated or absent parents. In obstetrics and pediatrics, both a child and her parents are in some sense patients. What should nurses who are committed to the radical dignity and equality of all human beings do when presented with conflicting interests?

Should a parent be given full authority to make health-care decisions—even if they are not in the best interest of the child? When is it right for health-care providers to intervene and override a parent's wishes?

One example of this was a case that Alisha had as a pediatric nurse in a children's hospital. She was taking care of a young child who, diagnosed with seizures as a toddler, was suffering greatly. No medications were able to effectively control his seizures. His parents, with the guidance of a neurologist from out of town, decided to trial the patient off medications and begin a ketogenic diet, which has been used for years for children with seizures. After stopping medications and starting the specialty diet, the child was admitted to the floor for breakthrough seizures. The parents refused medications because they wanted to trial the alternate approach. The pediatric hospitalist became increasingly frustrated with the parents and threatened to call Child Protective Services (CPS) unless they agreed to his recommended treatment. As a nurse, Alisha was torn on this case. The parents were very upset, and it was clear they cared deeply for their son and were following the guidance of another outside provider. Their plan was one that was supported by evidence. They felt their child was in a transition period and they expected a temporary increase in his seizures. In defense of the pediatric hospitalist, it was very difficult to watch this child have multiple seizures an hour knowing that this could be causing long-term damage. The parents ended up starting him on medications and CPS was never called. Was this the right decision? Did the parents have a right to refuse treatment or should CPS have been called? And what role should the nurse have played in this situation?

These are complicated questions that many nurses face when caring for the most vulnerable of patients. As mentioned previously, each of these next few chapters will have a particular focus on a single case study illustrating its central bioethical and theological concern. With that in mind, let us now shift our focus to a case in which human worth and equality are the central question—one of the most famous cases in all of bioethics—the case of Baby Doe.

CASE STUDY: BABY DOE

In 1982 an infant who became known as Baby Doe was born at a hospital in the Midwest. His case became well known and caused a public outcry at the time. Baby Doe was born with Trisomy 21, commonly known as Down syndrome. He was also born with tracheoesophageal fistula that made oral intake impossible and required surgical intervention in order for the child to take oral feedings.[10] The parents, who had two other "healthy" children, did not know of these conditions prior to delivery of Baby Doe.[11]

Tracheoesophageal fistula was then and remains now a fairly common issue for newborns who generally have a very good prognosis with surgery. The hospital at which Baby Doe was born at did not perform this type of surgery. The child's pediatrician recommended he be transferred to a pediatric hospital for surgical repair, which was common practice for the hospital when a child needed the surgery. However, the obstetrician had a different recommendation. Based on his vision of the good, he felt that non-intervention was the best option given the child's diagnosis of Down syndrome. This would result in the child dying of dehydration and starvation in a few days. It is important to understand that if the child was born only with the tracheoesophageal fistula and not Down syndrome, then this case never would have become a case at all. The physician and the hospital would have pushed for surgically repairing the defect since it is a fairly easy surgery with an excellent prognosis. But the obstetrician took the child's Down syndrome diagnosis and based his recommendation on what he felt was a life not worth living. He later testified that, "Even if surgery were successful, the possibility of minimally adequate quality of life was non-existent due to the child's severe and irreversible mental retardation."[12] The parents, in their state of shock and grief, decided to go with the obstetrician's recommendation and withhold treatment and allow the infant to die.

This decision caused an outraged response from other physicians, nurses, the hospital, and the community. The special-care nurses threatened to walk out of the hospital if the baby was not removed from the nursery. They struggled having to watch the newborn suffer. Their nursing—as well as their human—instincts to care and nurture were being threatened. Baby Doe was moved off of the floor into a private room where the parents were forced to hire private nurses to care for him.[13]

Hospital administrators and pediatricians created a legal case and an emergency court hearing was conducted.[14] The day after Baby Doe was born an emergency hearing was held at the hospital to determine whether the parents had a right to choose withholding treatment that would result in the death of their child. During the hearing, an attorney was present to represent the parents. However, no attorney was present to represent Baby Doe.[15] The court upheld the parents' right to refuse treatment. Two subsequent appeals were made on behalf of the child. There was an emergency appeal brought to the state's Supreme Court that was unsuccessful. Six days after Baby Doe was born, he died of dehydration and pneumonia while the guardian ad litem was on his way to Washington, DC, to appeal the case to the US Supreme Court.[16] There were several couples who petitioned to adopt Baby Doe and several petitioned to provide food and water temporarily to the child so that the case could be heard in the US Supreme Court. Those petitions fell on deaf ears.[17]

Throughout the six days that Baby Doe was alive, several attorneys attempted to intervene in the case. Three attorneys—Barry Brown, Lawrence Brodeur, and Philip Hill—decided to have the child declared neglected under Indiana's Child in Need of Services (CHINS) statute. They felt that allowing this case to move forward could set a frightening new precedent allowing parents who did not like their child to be able to end its life. Unfortunately for Baby Doe, the judge did not uphold the neglect charges since the Does were "following a medically recommended course of treatment for their child."[18] Many nurses disagreed with this decision. They felt the child was not only being neglected but was being treated inhumanely by being allowed to die a slow, painful death when a treatment was available. It was the nurses in the end who were there while Baby Doe took his last breath—his parents chose not to be there. It was the nurses who cradled him, wiped away his tears, and wiped his cracked, dehydrated mouth. And it was the nurses who wiped away his blood when his body started to hemorrhage freely through his nose and mouth as death became near.[19] And it was the nurses who—while helpless against the rulings—watched him take his last breath while the legal system and misguided obstetrician allowed such an awful plight for one of the most vulnerable patient populations—a newborn child.

HOW WE FAILED BABY DOE

How should Christians approach this case? Like most of the cases we will look at in each of these seven chapters, it involves more than one of our central principles. But the central principle at stake is obviously what we have been talking about above: human beings are made equal in the image and likeness of God. Baby Doe's obstetrician, as well as his own parents, viewed him as not worthy of life, and certainly not equal to the rest of us, due to his disability. This was an astonishingly evil judgment, one which was rightly condemned by the nurses and several physicians surrounding Baby Doe at the time, and one which has been judged as a gross example of ableism by almost everyone in bioethics classes for decades.

So that was a fundamental problem—Baby Doe's fundamental equality was rejected on the basis of his disability. But there are still more issues in play here. In several medical contexts, parents are given the right to choose the course of treatment for their child. In this case, the parents did in fact choose a treatment based at least in part on the advice and guidance of a provider. In other context, when parents and physicians agree, there can be times where treatment is forgone even if death is foreseen. For instance, parents may decide in a horribly tragic situation that further chemotherapy for their child with terminal cancer may be cruel and therefore choose to stop such treatment. In such a case, they are not aiming at the death of their child. In the best interests of their child, they are refusing to continue burdensome treatment that is not likely to have a positive effect. They are choosing to act in a way that *respected* the fundamentally equal dignity of their child. Indeed, if somehow their child miraculously recovered from the cancer even after stopping the chemotherapy they would be thrilled! Their goal was not to kill their child, but to spare her the pain of continued medical intervention.

This was not the case for Baby Doe. In this case, the parents and doctors decided that his life was not worth living and aimed at his death by omission of care. The repair of his esophagus was not painful nor burdensome. In refusing this medical treatment the goal was clear: that Baby Doe would die because it was better that someone with his disability die than live. If Baby Doe had somehow lived (say, if the nurses were sneaking nutrition to him through an IV or gastrostomy tube [G-tube]) the parents and doctors would not have been thrilled. On the contrary, they would have been quite upset at having their goal thwarted here.

Unfortunately, during the time of the Baby Doe case it was not uncommon for physicians to have similar views of disabled children as the obstetrician who encouraged the parents to withhold treatment and allow their child to die. A 1973 article published in *The New England Journal of Medicine* discussed the fact that babies were often allowed to die. The researchers reviewed nearly three hundred infant deaths over a two-year period and found that 14 percent were related to withholding treatment. The authors strongly endorsed joint decisions made by both physicians and families to withhold treatment. Furthermore, they noted that some families cited their reason for withholding treatment was based on the perceived burden of raising a disabled child.[20] However, one year later David Smith, an ethics professor, published a very different view in medical ethics literature. He argued that "the only fair criterion for deciding appropriate treatment for a given baby is that baby's own welfare and ability to receive love."[21] Smith's criterion seems to fit more with a Christian view of pediatric ethics.

Another important consideration is the ability of parents to make these complex decisions directly after birth. When parents are presented with the news that their child is diagnosed with abnormalities, they are often understandably met with feelings of shock, fear, guilt, shame, and grief. And this can last for months.[22] Furthermore, parents often lack the information to make informed decisions and often underestimate the potential of the child. Parents are vulnerable to the suggestions of health-care providers with an ableist view about quality of life. Some note that parents are understandably concerned with potentially devastating effects on their family from social, financial, and psychological perspectives.[23] This is where Christian nurses can play a key role, helping parents who seem overwhelmed (understandably) by the gravity of the moment to see more clearly how to respect fundamental human dignity and equality. Nurses will be able to bring their broad experience to bear and let parents know, for instance, about the stories of others who have been in similar situations.

All health-care providers—but especially those claimed by Christ—have a duty to protect the most vulnerable. Baby Doe, a voiceless child who could not speak for himself, saw those who had power over him decide that his disabled life was not worth living. This, despite the fact that his nurses fought for him and several families stepped up to be his caretakers and adopt him. He was still denied life—indeed, those who were supposed to care for him instead aimed at his death—because of his perceived disability.

THE RIGHT AND DUTY TO STAND UP

Unfortunately, similar cases with similar moral reasoning to this still occur to this day. There are tragic times in a neonatal intensive care unit (NICU), or in a nursing home, when family and physicians aim at the death of certain disabled human beings who are deemed "less than" other human beings. Someone might have had a severe congenital malformation in utero—or maybe a person develops substantial dementia. Or maybe there is some other scenario in which a particular human being is deemed "less than" another and refused the same kind of treatment and care.

In the specific case of Baby Doe, the nurses at the hospital were ultimately limited in what they could have done. Alisha can empathize with their situation, having worked in a children's hospital as a nurse, caring for vulnerable children. She felt the impact of the case personally. As a pediatric nurse and an adoptive mother to a child born with medical concerns, she has witnessed severely conflicting opinions on what is considered to be in the "best interest" of those vulnerable children. She feels fortunate that most of the nurses and physicians she worked with were Christian and believed that each child had inherent worth and deserved dignity and love. Caring for the pediatric patients would have been immeasurably more difficult had her colleagues' moral compasses been so different that they could not, at the very least, agree on those truths.

The nurses caring for Baby Doe were not as fortunate. Though they spoke up strongly in the beginning, once the legal process began, they were bound by legal decisions that were made. Many of the nurses rightly refused to take part in his treatment since they could not just sit back and watch a newborn child die without intervening, and as a result they provide an inspiring example for nurses today. We will look at conscientious refusal and its protection—along with the proper role nurses ought to have on medical teams—in later chapters. But here it may be important simply to say that nurses today are in a much different position than nurses of the 1980s. Nurses today can call ethics consultants. Nurses today are considered (or ought to be considered) full-fledged members of the medical team, members who have the right and the duty to stand up and let their voices be heard. Christian nurses today should follow the example of the nurses from the Baby Doe case in standing up for the dignity of all human beings created equal in the divine image.

DISCUSSION QUESTIONS

1. How would you describe what was done to Baby Doe? Is killing an appropriate description? Why or why not?
2. What role should Christian nurses have played in the case of Baby Doe? What specific steps would you have taken were you part of the medical team?
3. Prenatal children are killed at very high rates via abortion in most Western countries.[24] Do you see any connection between this practice and what went on in the Baby Doe case?
4. The relationship between parents and members of the health-care team can be complex in thinking about what is best for a child, especially if they have different visions of the good. What does the Baby Doe case teach us about how those relationships should work?

6

FROM FERTILIZATION TO NATURAL DEATH

When you see someone's sacredness, everything changes.

– Barbara Lynn Vannoy

In the previous chapter we discussed human worth and human dignity. God has created all human beings with a nature that bears His image and likeness and it is in sharing this common nature that all of us are fundamentally equal. Our role as health-care providers should be to care for all human beings with this kind of equality in mind, regardless of their particular genetic makeup or capacities. But two significant questions of bioethics now present themselves: (1) when does one of these fundamentally equal human beings come into existence and (2) when does one go out of existence? This chapter will seek to answer both these questions by looking deeper at the second key theological principle: a particular human being is identical to a particular living human organism. Though we have an essential spiritual component, we are fundamentally living bodies who begin our existence as human organisms after fertilization and end our existence when our human body dies.

NURSING CARE FOR ALL LIVING HUMAN BEINGS

There are a wide range of health-care contexts in which nurses are faced with the question of when human life begins and when it ends: obstetrics (especially abortion), fertility medicine, neonatal treatment and care, intensive care (especially when a patient has a catastrophic brain injury), organ transplant teams, and more. Christian nurses come into their job with particular commitments to fundamental human equality in ways that can have a dramatic impact as to how they approach each of these health-care contexts. In addition, it is important to be aware of potential ethical situations you might find yourself in and form an understanding and belief of what is the most Christ-like response. This is important for all members of the health-care team to do. Here is a section taken from the Biblical Model for Medical Ethics written by Christian Medical and Dental Associations:

> The circumstances of each case must be considered to discover the moral issues raised, but we do not accept such philosophies as ethical relativism, situational ethics, or utilitarianism. Neither do we follow mindless legalism. Our Lord stated that the weightier matters of the law are justice, mercy, and faith in God. Biblical ethics is concerned with motives as well as actions, with process as well as outcome. The integrity of moral decisions rests on the prudent use of biblical principles. We acknowledge, however, that sincere Christians may differ in their interpretation and application of these principles. Patients or their advocates, families, and clinicians are morally responsible for their own actions. We, as physicians and dentists, are ultimately responsible to God as we care for the health of our fellow human beings.[1]

The stated goal of this book is to help each current or future nurse navigate through some of these ethical questions, to help you form your own belief that is founded in Christian theology, and to live out your calling morally and justly. We go through our day looking at situations through a medical lens. But how important it is to also consider things through a spiritual one.

There have been many cases over the years that really made Alisha step back and evaluate her own beliefs and question what truly was the morally correct course for a patient. And at no time in her profession was this more apparent than when she was working in a children's hospital (caring for newborns, children with disabilities, and children dying of cancer) and while working in a clinic with high-risk pregnancies. There were tragic cases, frankly, when she didn't see any good options. It was during those times that Alisha prayed deeply to have spiritual truths and a spiritual lens guide the moral compass she was using to navigate these cases.

There might be times where you will be faced with hard decisions regarding the care of unborn children or patients who are in a severely depressed level of consciousness. You might be in a position where you are caring for a pregnant mother who is struggling with addiction, became pregnant as a result of rape, or a mother who is struggling with whether to continue her pregnancy. How do you approach these situations? Nurses get lots of opinions and advice thrown their way during these times. There will also be moments where you might feel torn between your role as a nurse and your role as a Christian. Should a nurse, or any health-care worker, be forced to participate in procedures or treatment that go against their religious beliefs—abortion, for example? What about following through with an order that you know could result in the death or harm of a patient? Future chapters will focus on some of the legal and other issues involved in those questions, but for now, we are focusing just on the moral analysis. And with that in mind, let us dive right into a case study that, in some ways, could not more perfectly highlight what is at stake in determining when a new, fundamentally equal human being comes into existence and when one goes out of existence.

CASE STUDY: *MUÑOZ V. JOHN PETER SMITH HOSPITAL*

Erick Muñoz and Marlise Muñoz were a married couple and parents to a toddler. On November 26, 2013, while Marlise was approximately 14 weeks pregnant, she woke up in the middle of the night to make her son a bottle. About an hour later her husband went out into the kitchen and found her lying on the floor unconscious. She was rushed to John Peter Smith Hospital and it was determined that she collapsed from what they believed was a pulmonary embolism. On November 28, 2013, two days after she was found unresponsive, physicians declared Marlise brain-dead.[2]

Marlise and her husband Erick were both paramedics and had previous discussions of their wishes in the event they suffered medical emergencies. According to Erick, Marlise had expressed to him that in the event of brain death, she would not want to be kept alive artificially.[3] Her husband, wanting to respect her previously stated wishes, asked that she be removed from life support. Her other family was in support of this decision.[4] The hospital refused to grant their request, citing Section 166.049 of the Texas Health and Safety Code as the basis for their refusal.[5] This law required lifesaving measures to be maintained for pregnant patients, regardless if the patient had provided written or verbal wishes against lifesaving measures pre-pregnancy. They believed it was necessary to continue providing treatment since the fetus was still alive. However, it was later determined that the law only applies to patients who are considered alive and not for patients who are no longer living.[6] The refusal of the hospital to remove life support prompted Mr. Muñoz to file suit against John Peter Smith Hospital.[7]

The case continued for weeks while Mrs. Muñoz was kept alive on life support. Then in January 2014, the attorney representing Erick Muñoz cited that the continuing life support was not in alignment with the law since the mother was declared legally dead and the infant, while still alive, was suspected to be not viable. He made the argument that the unborn child appeared to have suffered from oxygen deprivation and had several medical effects, including extremity deformities, hydrocephalus, and a potential heart condition.[8] The court ruled that Section 166.049 of the Texas Health and Safety Code does not apply to patients who have been medically declared brain-dead and ordered the hospital to remove all life-sustaining equipment. On January 26, 2014, the hospital removed Mrs. Muñoz from life support. The baby, who was twenty-two weeks old at the time, died as a result.[9]

TWO LIVING HUMAN BEINGS

The *Muñoz v. John Peter Smith Hospital* case is fairly complicated. While this case highlights the key principle of this chapter—that human beings are living bodies and begin their existence as human organisms after fertilization—it also touches on a few other key principles.

Let us first look at the importance of fertilization. Most scientists agree that the life of a new human organism begins at fertilization. Fertilization involves the fusion of a spermatozoon and an oocyte, which becomes a zygote. This zygote is the beginning of a human being.[10] As O'Rahilly and Müller wrote in *Human Embryology and Teratology* in 1996: "Although human life is a continuous process, fertilization is a critical landmark because, under ordinary circumstances, a new, genetically distinct human organism is thereby formed. . . .The combination of 23 chromosomes present in each pronucleus results in 46 chromosomes in the zygote. Thus the diploid number is restored and the embryonic genome is formed. The embryo now exists as a genetic unity."[11]

The process of fertilization produces life. Some argue that a zygote is not a human, but rather a collection of cells, brought forth by the spermatozoon and oocyte. However, this is not accurate when you look at it from a biological, science-centered perspective. A zygote is merely the first stage in the development of a distinct human organism. As Austriaco observed, "The earliest two-celled mammalian embryo is a two-celled individual and not two individual cells."[12] Different stages of development do not change the fact that one is more "human" at different stages. Villanova University philosophy professor Dr. Stephen Napier provides a unique way to understand this: "A corollary of the idea that organisms grow and develop is that an organism preserves its identity through changes. Thus, there are phases of one and the same entity: zygote, morula, blastocyst, embryo, fetus, neonate, infant, toddler, and so forth. This may be a picayune observation to some, but these are treacherous waters wherein confusion threatens. The confusion concerns levels of identity. Identity is always specific to a sort or category. I am the same human being as I was, when I was a boy; but I am not identical to the boy I was simply because I am no longer a boy."[13] This is a beautiful way to look at a fetus, as a distinct human in the process of transition—and if nature allows, will continue to transition through stages into adulthood. Isn't that what being alive is really about—a series of transitions and transformations from life to death?

And what about death? What is the Christian viewpoint of when death occurs? Pope Saint John Paul II, while answering this question, stated, "This gives rise to one of the most debated issues in contemporary bioethics, as well as to serious concerns in the minds of ordinary people. I refer to the problem of *ascertaining the fact of death*. When can a person be considered dead with complete certainty?"[14] From a Christian perspective, human death is the separation of the soul from the body. John Haas writes in the *National Catholic Bioethics Quarterly* in 2011, "The reason no scientific technique can directly identify the moment of death is quite simple: the soul is a non-corporeal, spiritual life-principle which cannot be observed or measured or weighed using the tools of empirical science. The presence or absence of the soul can be ascertained only by observing certain biological signs that indirectly attest to its presence or its absence."[15] Pope Saint Paul II further discusses the moment of death as it relates to the medical determination of death: "The death of the person . . . is an event which no scientific technique or empirical method can identify directly. Yet human experience shows that once death occurs certain biological signs inevitably follow, which medicine has learnt to recognize with increasing precision. In this sense, the 'criteria' for ascertaining death used by medicine today should not be understood as the technical-scientific determination of the exact moment of a person's death, but as a scientifically secure means of identifying the biological signs that a person has indeed died."[16]

While there is no clear way to measure the exact moment when someone passes, medicine has some criteria that is used to declare someone legally dead. In the past, death was defined as the cessation of the heart beating. However, someone's heart can stop beating and still live if the heart begins beating again. The definition of death, at least in most circles, now involves the brain. The medical declaration of brain death is defined as "the permanent loss of function of the entire brain, including the brain stem."[17] With this definition, there is no reversing brain death. This is different than a patient being considered comatose or in a vegetative state. When a patient is in a coma, they have a severely depressed level of consciousness, but not irreversible loss of all brain function. When a patient is in a vegetative state, he or she often has continued function of the brainstem, which allows them to continue vital functions. When a patient is declared brain-dead, he or she has complete and irreversible loss of all brain function.[18] Theologically speaking, there is no consensus as to an exact moment when the body and spirit separate.

In the above case study, there are two living human beings—the mother and the unborn child. As stated above, Marlise Muñoz was declared brain-dead. However, she—which we established in the previous chapter—is a living organism, and that organism is still very much alive. Her other organs are working in a systematic way with her body maintaining homeostasis. She is fighting off infections and when she suffers trauma her heart rate goes up and adrenaline is released. And of course, she is nourishing and gestating her baby. The issue with this case is that there are two humans involved, each with their own God-given dignity and equality.

But what about a mother who is considered brain-dead, as in the case of Marlise Muñoz? She had rights and even stated her desires about not wanting to be on life support with her family prior to her tragic event. But no one could have truly known if her wish to not be on life support included while pregnant, since this conversation did not take place. Even if she did have this conversation, does her desire not to be kept alive outweigh the child's right to life? In this case, it is important to weigh the autonomy of a brain-dead woman against the interests of a living fetus.

Margaret Somerville, founding director of McGill University's Centre for Medicine, Ethics and Law in Montréal, Quebec, argues that "You've got the potential of major benefit to the unborn child if it survives and very little downside to keeping [the mother] on life support until you could deliver the baby at a reasonable time."[19] In the case of Muñoz, many argue that the child may face death or disability anyway, and this could lead to financial burden to the family. Somerville has argued, "What you're saying is that being dead is better than having a life that involves disability or suffering."[20] Again, this can be a dangerous conclusion to make—one that can be abused in cases where the best interest of the patient is not at the forefront.

Though this varies around the world, in most rich Western nations prenatal children are not thought of as being the same as older children. Or, if they are, it is because they are wanted rather than unwanted. We see this with the importance of language. Physicians and nurses use the term "baby" when talking to a pregnant woman about her wanted prenatal child, saying things like, "Let's check your baby's heart rate," or "You should feel the baby kick." It would feel out of place if one said, "You should feel your fetus kick." We use this language outside of a health-care setting as well. We throw a mother-to-be a "baby shower" rather than a "fetus shower." We comment on her "baby bump." Such clinical language is used to play up the equal humanity of the baby when wanted, but not when she is not wanted. This violates, clearly, a Christian understanding of dignity and equality.

We already discussed one concept of the start of life—stages of development and identity. This is just one argument made by individuals who do not view unborn children as a "person" with fundamental rights. An embryo is not identical to an adult, correct, but this does not change the fact that it is still the same human, just at a different stage. An embryo will later become an infant, then a toddler, then eventually an adult. Same person, different stages. But as we've discussed at other points in this book, another argument commonly made in situations like this is that in order for a human to exist, there must be developed psychological capacities.[21] This is an argument we covered in the previous chapter when discussing the case of Baby Doe. Again, this argument quickly falls apart once one realizes that certain circumstances make it difficult, even impossible, to continue with this view. If psychological capacity is the determining factor for being declared human, then what happens when psychological capacity is compromised? Is someone no longer a human if they are in a coma, on the operating table, or sleeping? Is a toddler less human than an adult? What about an elderly patient who suffers from dementia? See where this can get murky? Having a belief and understanding that a human becomes a human at fertilization, unlike the other cases, does not change with circumstances, disabilities, or stages of life. Fertilization creates a unique human with forty-six chromosomes. Period.

A CONFLICT OF RIGHTS?

Jesus, of course, never speaks of rights—and certainly not about rights in the way we tend to do in the developed West. Still, most reading these pages in our culture are understandably drawn to ask about the rights of the mother in this case. Our main goal in this chapter is to focus on when a human being comes into existence and when they die, but one could also ask whether a mother's rights outweigh the rights of her unborn child. This is a massive question, one that goes beyond the scope of what we are up to in this chapter. But in thinking about it, let's consider a case that happened in Indiana back in 2013. An infant estimated to be 25 weeks gestation, well beyond the age at which babies survive outside their mother's body, was found dead in a dumpster behind a restaurant. The child was determined to be that of a Purvi Patel, whose family owned the restaurant. She had purchased abortive medications over the internet and induced an abortion. She stated the baby was stillborn at the time of delivery, but the autopsy showed that the baby did take at least one breath. Purvi stated that she believed she was only about 10–12 weeks pregnant at the time of the abortion. She was arrested for the abortion and the death of her infant son.[22]

During the trial, prosecutors pushed for Purvi to receive forty years in prison. She was sentenced to twenty years in prison for charges of feticide as well as neglect, since she did not seek medical care for her child, who was born alive. Purvi appealed the sentence based on what her attorneys felt was a misinterpretation of the feticide law. They argued that Indiana's feticide law wasn't meant to be used to prosecute women for their own abortions. In 2016 her sentence was overturned and Purvi was released from prison.[23] If Purvi were to have walked into an abortion clinic and paid for a legal abortion, then she would not have been prosecuted for the death of her child. The killing of an unborn child is legal as long as it is done within sterile white walls by a professional. But, at least for the Indiana prosecutors, it is wrong if it is done at home by the mother.

In thinking about the "conflict of rights" between a mother and her child, it is first incredibly important to attend to what moral theologians and philosophers call "the anthropology" (a vision of the human person) right at a foundational level. As is by now clear from this chapter and the previous one, pregnancy involves a unique relationship between two human beings made in the image and likeness of God. And, again, that is our main focus in this chapter. Beyond that, in order to conclude anything about the morality (or say nothing of legality) of abortion itself would go well beyond the scope of this chapter. (Charlie has written a book titled *Beyond the Abortion Wars* if readers want to get into the complexity.[24]) We don't think "conflict of rights" is the best tool for expressing right relationships between human beings made in the image and likeness of God. Even so, theologian and pastor John Piper used a helpful analogy to think about it using the secular language of our time: "We know the principle of justice that when two legitimate rights conflict, the right that protects the higher value should prevail. We deny the right to drive at 100 miles per hour because the value of life is greater than the value of being on time or getting thrills. The right of the unborn not to be killed and the right of a woman not to be pregnant may be at odds. But they are not equal rights. Staying alive is more precious and more basic than not being pregnant."[25]

While this is true, it still leaves several questions unanswered about the moral and legal questions surrounding the act of abortion. Our opponents on this issue, for instance, sometimes describe attempts to make abortion illegal as something like forced slavery of the woman in service of the fetus. They note that even if the fetus is a human being, fathers are not forced to donate non-vital organs to their children (like a kidney) even if their child will die without it. So why is a woman forced to use her body to support a fetus?

Perhaps the most famous article ever written on abortion was by a philosopher, Judith Jarvis Thomson.[26] For the sake of argument only, she gives pro-lifers the fact that the fetus is a human being (she doesn't agree) but then offers the following thought experiment to justify her pro-choice position. Suppose you were whisked way in the middle of the night by the Society of Professional Music Lovers and, using a new technology, they attached you to the body of a famous violinist they want to be kept alive. When you wake up, obviously startled and in distress, they say you just have to stay attached to the violinist for a few months while they find a suitable kidney donor. Thomson then asks us if we have the right to remove ourselves from the violinist—foreseeing that he will die if we do. She then builds on the intuition that most will say something like "yes, while it may be a good thing to stay attached, it is not killing a legitimate choice to remove one's self from the violinist" to draw the analogy to abortion. A woman disconnecting herself from the fetus is not killing the child and, using Piper's "hierarchy of rights" language right back at him, the right of the woman not to be enslaved in bodily service to another trumps the right of another person to have another person sustain them with their body.

One can see how complex these questions can get. (And this doesn't even address what can be reasonably done via the law.) Thomson's argument has generated a tremendous amount of response literature and it goes beyond the scope of this chapter to respond to it here. However, we will say two things. First, Thomson's analogy might work for rare examples where abortion is sought as response to pregnancy as a result of sexual violence, but not other kinds of pregnancy. Consensual sex, as everyone who has taken middle school science knows, is at least in part ordered to procreation and pregnancy. Those are just stubborn facts of biology.

Second, and here we transition into the topic of the next chapter, most abortions are much more like direct killings rather than nonviolent removals of someone from one's body. Indeed, in most abortion circumstances (like the incredibly high rate of abortion in the case of children with Down syndrome[27]) the goal is not simply to remove a child from one's body, but to actually kill a human being. And so, this is another sense in which most abortion circumstances don't work with Thomson's famous analogy. The vast majority of abortions are attempts to kill, not merely choices not to aid or to "let die."

The distinction between killing and letting die, not least because it comes up in so many areas of medicine, is an absolutely crucial one in medical ethics. And it is to this topic we turn in the next chapter.

DISCUSSION QUESTIONS

1. Pregnancy is described in this chapter as involving two living human beings. Many people take issue with describing the prenatal child as a human being. What beliefs do you hold (biological, theological, moral, and so on) that shape your opinion on whether pregnancy involves two living human beings or just one?
2. What kinds of social structures would have to be in place in order to foster a culture that protects vulnerable, prenatal children and their mothers?
3. What role can nurses play—whether through advocacy or in the workplace—in being a voice for vulnerable, both prenatal children and their mothers?
4. Does it make sense to describe a human female body that is successfully gestating her prenatal child as dead? What implications does your answer have for the current use of brain death as a coherent standard for death?
5. All nurses are confronted with death. How are your views about death informed by your Christian faith? How might you see death in a way that is different from your non-Christian colleagues and patients?

7

ACCEPTING DEATH, NEVER KILLING

> Survival is the celebration of choosing life over death. We know we're going to die. We all die. But survival is saying: perhaps not today. In that sense, survivors don't defeat death, they come to terms with it.
>
> – *Laurence Gonzales*

In the previous chapter, we left off thinking about the distinction between killing and letting die. This distinction calls to mind the principle which will be the focus of this chapter: Accept death when it comes without violently aiming at it. Here once again we imitate the example of our Lord himself who defeated death only after a refusal to resist a humiliating and terrible crucifixion. Christians do not avoid death at all costs but rather come to accept it as a natural part of life. Like Jesus our master, we do not aim at our own deaths or the deaths of others. He did not aim at his own death—indeed, His agony in the Garden of Gethsemane and prayer to the Father that the cup would pass from Him indicates this quite clearly. Christians are forbidden from engaging in this kind of violence as a fundamental attack on the God-given dignity of the human person made in the divine image. Our lives ultimately belong to our Creator, not to us. God is the Lord of life and death. We are not.

But isn't there a kind of tension here? Especially in a time when so many think of ethics in terms of consequentialist utilitarianism, many may see killing vs. accepting death as a distinction without a moral difference. Don't both scenarios end up with someone dead at the end of the day? But as we also discussed in chapter 4, a Christian theological vision insists on distinguishing between two very morally different actions (or omissions): (1) those which in their very natures attack the goodness and dignity of the human life and (2) those which acknowledge its goodness and dignity and, while foreseeing and allowing death, don't aim at it. A good death for one of our fellow human beings is one in which we stand firm in our supernatural hope while refusing to abandon the dignity and present needs of the still living patient, especially via palliative and spiritual care. We help our brother or sister in Christ choose how to live out their final days without choosing to snuff out their life as worthless. Though we accept the reality of death, this is perhaps the most important time to be lovingly present to everyone involved—especially given that our death-denying culture can make facing the truth of our ultimate destiny that much more difficult.

NOT KILLING, BUT ACCEPTING DEATH IN NURSING

Nurses in nearly every field of medicine are confronted with how to handle the end of life: from the emergency room, home care, critical care units, surgery, labor and delivery, neonatal intensive care, geriatrics, nursing homes, and even outpatient settings. Death is something nurses spend years learning how to help patients avoid. Mirroring our broader culture, the word "death" is often taboo in health care. On some level we know that death is just as natural a part of life as birth is, but losing a patient is not easy. And while we have come a long way in understanding end-of-life care, this is an area that is still needing more focus. The Institute of Medicine highlighted this in a report put out in 2015. The authors wrote:

> At present, the U.S. health care system is ill designed to meet the needs of patients near the end of life and their families. The system is geared to providing acute care aimed at curing disease, but not at providing the comfort care most people near end of life prefer. The financial incentives built into the programs that most often serve people with advanced serious illnesses—Medicare and Medicaid— are not well coordinated, and the result is fragmented care that increases risks to patients and creates avoidable burdens on them and their families.[1]

Not surprisingly, nurses often struggle with several moral questions when caring for patients during end-of-life care. One might be concerned with administering opioid analgesics for comfort, knowing that it also acts as a respiratory depressant, potentially hastening death.[2] Or a nurse might question the withholding or withdrawing of treatment, such as nutrition, fluids, or medication. The order for withholding or withdrawing can come from either a physician or the patients themselves. It can be difficult to care for a patient who refuses potential lifesaving treatment. For instance, a patient who is tired of fighting cancer and requests all chemotherapeutics be stopped. Or a daughter who requests life support be removed from her elderly father who suffered a stroke. Is there a difference between never starting treatment or stopping it once it has been started? According to the American Nurses Association, "Providers should never start a therapy they are not willing to discontinue."[3] Which of these are examples of aiming to kill someone? Which are examples of helping a patient choose how to live out their final days? Even for many Christian nurses, allowing death to occur can feel equivalent to killing, while for others it may feel quite different. This chapter will attempt to sort out the reasoning.

Though we will look at this kind of case in detail later in the book, it is also worth mentioning here. Another common dilemma nurses face when caring for patients nearing death is the often-conflicting role of caring for the needs of both the patient and the family. Each person, obviously, experiences death differently and many have different lenses and values they use to make sense of it. For some, death is unexpected and tragic; for others death might bring an end to a long battle filled with suffering.[4] In addition, some of the patients experience a long illness which allows them to be part of the treatment decision-making process. For others, illness is sudden, and families are given the responsibility of decision-making on behalf of the patient. But what should a nurse do when family members don't agree on the care plan, or when families struggle with accepting death when it is inevitable? During these times, the nurse has an incredible responsibility to navigate each case delicately, wisely, and with intent to provide compassionate care to both the patient and the family.

As mentioned, we will discuss precisely this kind of situation in a future chapter—one which employs a Trinitarian vision that tries to honor both the dignity of the individual and dignity of the communal/familial. But, for now, let us turn to a particular case study that directly highlights what is at stake in the central moral-theological principle in the chapter.

CASE STUDY: MURDER OR MERCY? THE CASE OF DR. WILLIAM HUSEL

On November 13, 2018, a twenty-seven-year-old registered nurse named Stephanie found herself in an uncomfortable position many nurses can relate to. She had started working at a new hospital, Mount Carmel, just a few months prior to the case in question. She was working in the intensive care unit (ICU), a new area for her, and caring for an eighty-year-old female patient who suffered a cardiac arrest and was struggling to breathe.[5] This was Stephanie's first end-of-life case. The ICU physician in charge that night, Dr. William Husel, ordered Stephanie to give the patient 1,000 mcg of Fentanyl for comfort measures. This is a much higher dose than typically seen on other units. Stephanie asked two separate colleagues about this dose; she was assured that this was Dr. Husel's standard of care. She went ahead and gave the Fentanyl dose and within twenty-three minutes of receiving the medication, the patient died. Eight days later, Mount Carmel Health systems fired Dr. Husel.[6] This was not an isolated case: Dr. Husel was being accused of overmedicating multiple patients, resulting in the deaths of dozens of his patients. Stephanie would later find out that she was one of thirty-five employees who were either put on administrative leave or fired. The hospital accused nurses and pharmacists of not catching or reporting the excessive doses of Fentanyl, filling the prescriptions (pharmacists), or following through with medication administration (nurses). Throughout the investigation, forty-eight employees were reported to their respective boards, and twenty-five nurses risked losing their licenses.[7]

The investigation of Dr. Husel is still ongoing at the time our book goes to press. He has been portrayed in two very different lights—as both a caring physician who was providing treatment out of compassion and a physician who misused medications for the purpose of hastening death. Since the hospital began investigating these cases of overmedication, Dr. Husel has been charged with the murder of twenty-five patients. Most of them were being given care at the very end of their lives as they were weaned from life support. While there is no set maximum dose for Fentanyl for these types of cases, any dose greater than 500 mcg could be considered lethal.[8] In the twenty-five cases where Dr. Husel is being charged with murder, patients received 500–2,000 mcg per dose. There are cases where patients received higher doses that did not result in death, and Dr. Husel has argued that he was working within his scope of acceptable practice to provide comfort to patients during their final moments. Robert Landy, a lawyer representing several former employees who have filed charges against the hospital, stated, "The compassionate very-end-of-life care that the 35 patients received had a single goal: to allow them to die with dignity and without pain in accordance with their families' wishes."[9]

While the fate of Dr. Husel awaits his trial, this case provides a look into the balance that many nurses face when providing end-of-life care—making sure patients are comfortable, following through with provider orders, and practicing safe and effective care. Nurses play pivotal roles in helping patients die comfortably and with dignity. Nurses must use their assessment skills to evaluate whether patients are in pain and advocate when there appears to be avoidable suffering. Pain medications can help relieve suffering, but high doses can also result in respiratory depression. The particular case here involving Dr. Husel and his staff helps us get at the heart of the important distinction between accepting death and never killing.

WHAT WAS DR. HUSEL'S INTENT?

Certain acts, especially when looked at via Christian ethics, are going to be wrong no matter what they intend. Aiming at the death of an innocent person is always wrong, for instance, even when one wants to bring about a good outcome. Christians are not utilitarians who think that all that matters is producing good consequences. On the contrary, we believe that we are beholden to the commands of God and that it is His job to make sure things come out right, not ours. Again, God is the Lord of life and we are not. This prohibits every kind of aiming at the death of a patient via euthanasia or assisted suicide. Christian nurses should refuse to participate in the kind of violence which is the antithesis of health care.

But the case of Dr. Husel provides an interesting, complex, and significant story for us to examine. It is significant here in this chapter because it can show us that not all actions which accept the reality of death and focus on a way someone wishes to live are necessarily examples of killing. To be clear, and this is what makes this kind of case complex, if Dr. Husel was trying to kill these patients near the end of their lives he may have performed exactly the same kind of *physical* action: prescribing very high doses of Fentanyl. But moral actions like giving someone pain medication can't be reduced to their physical description—Dr. Husel's intention is key for making a moral evaluation of what he and his staff did here. It is possible that he intended to kill these patients as a means of saving them from suffering at the very end of their lives. But this is euthanasia—taking the life of the patient into our hands as if it belongs to us—which is never acceptable because it misunderstands our relationship to our Creator. On the contrary, it is also possible that Dr. Husel gave this very high dose because he thought it was the kind of dose necessary to control their pain and he *merely foresaw* but did *not* intend to kill.

If he had the latter intent, then he is in the moral clear. Again, Christians (and most other folks) are not consequentialists: almost everyone understands that there is a major moral distinction, for instance, between plans for military bombing runs which attempt to avoid but nevertheless foresee some civilian deaths and plans for bombing runs which *intend* the deaths of civilians. We have no right to intend and use the death of another for our own purposes. That kind of act is proper to the Lord of life and death alone. There are perfectly moral (though often tragic) actions, by contrast, in which one doesn't intend someone's death but sees that it is likely to happen. During the COVID-19 pandemic, for instance, we became quite familiar with another dilemma like this: allocating mechanical ventilators when the need was greater than the supply.[10] When in such a desperate situation, the choice to allocate ventilators for some patients—while foreseeing that some patients will not get them (and likely die)—is not the same as a choice to kill. Far from it.

If a health-care provider like Dr. Husel is intending to control pain—with a focus on helping a patient live a certain way (as pain-free as possible)—then the fact that he may also foresee (but not intend) that death may come faster than it otherwise would, can justify his action.

WORRIES ABOUT A SLIPPERY SLOPE

It can be difficult to determine someone's intention, especially in a health-care context. One technique Charlie sometimes uses with his students is to do a thought experiment in which the patient unexpectedly lives and think about what the reaction of the health-care provider would be. Suppose in one of the cases where Dr. Husel gave the large dose of pain medication the patient unexpectedly started breathing after being removed from the ventilator. Would he be upset or not? If upset, it seems his goal was to kill the patient given that this goal was thwarted. If not upset, then it seems his goal was not to kill the patient as the goal to control pain was achieved without death taking place.

There is a concern, however, that in part because intention can be complex and difficult to discern that these practices can lead to a slippery slope toward normalizing assisted suicide and euthanasia. After all, as we highlighted in chapter 5, major injustices in health care tend to have small beginnings. Some, for instance, believe with good reason that palliative sedation—in which one with intense pain in the dying process, though not killed, is kept unconscious on their way to death—is an excellent alternative to aiming at their death.[11] But it is relatively easy to slide from this into using medication simply to keep patients "docile" when they are difficult to care for—a practice that is relatively common now in nursing homes, particularly when a patient has dementia.[12]

The complexity and gray areas that sometimes accompany these kinds of shifts, though they may seem small and inconsequential, may in fact be the small beginnings of much larger moral problems—like the widespread push for direct killing via assisted suicide and euthanasia that has gained such momentum in recent years. And, if we are generous, the discussion above might help us understand the impulse to move in this direction. The fact that the *same exact physical act* performed by Dr. Husel (say, prescribing someone 1,000 mcg of Fentanyl) could be either praised as compassionate or condemned as murder could easily become confusing to someone who hasn't thought about these issues very deeply. Indeed, it may be totally unclear even on what basis one could claim a moral line has been crossed simply based on something that one cannot see in the physical world: a moral agent's intention.

The key is to hold onto the duty of the Christian and the healthcare provider to also provide care and never to kill. A duty to help one's patients *live a certain way*, even through the process of their dying, and not to snuff out their life. Significantly for this discussion, good palliative care and good care for the general well-being of patients at the end of their lives obviates most requests for assisted suicide. Again, given the busyness of most physicians, the role of making patients understand that they are valued often falls to nurses. If dying patients can be reassured their life has meaning, that they are personally valued and loved, hospice directors find that their residents don't request assisted suicide. Indeed, in the state of Oregon (which has had legalized assisted suicide for the longest time of any US state) requests for death because of physical pain and suffering don't even make the top five reasons offered. Far more central to such requests are social issues like fear of being a burden on others.[13] The kind of caring for the whole person described throughout this book as central to an understanding of Christian nursing becomes absolutely essential here if we are to resist a culture that would rather discard patients than encounter them in a spirit of loving hospitality.

OTHER KINDS OF CASES

The first reaction many of our students have to the kind of reasoning used above is to consider it a kind of "cheating" in one's moral reasoning. A way of justifying killing without admitting that you are killing. This, from our perspective, is the fruit of the deep influence that utilitarian consequentialism has had on both contemporary health care and Western culture in general. To reiterate: from military ethics to the allocation of scarce medical resources, almost all of us understand quite intuitively that not every action in which we can foresee death as a likely consequence is like killing. Or even *at all* like killing. This reasoning has the kinds of implications discussed above when it comes to palliative care (as opposed to assisted suicide and euthanasia), but it also has implications in many other areas of health care.

How should we describe, for instance, the withdrawal or withholding of a ventilator when there is no scarcity? Or the withdrawal or withholding of nutrition and hydration? How about discontinuing chemotherapeutics treating advanced-stage cancer? Refusing surfactant or other aggressive treatment of a baby in the NICU? While there are some morally relevant differences between these kinds of cases that go beyond the scope of this chapter, they often do connect to the central insight over accepting death while never killing. In many of these kinds of cases, the withdrawal or withholding may in fact be aiming at death. We saw this already in the case of Baby Doe in chapter 5: in that case, the physician and parents aimed at the death of their child by omission. One could also presumably aim at the death of a patient by omission in any of the examples above as well. But, as with the case of Dr. Husel, one may well have a very different intent. Given the discussion of Judith Jarvis Thomson's argument at the end of chapter 6, it is also worth noting here that this reasoning could also apply to whether an abortion of pregnancy is aiming at the death of the child or much more like removing the violinist.

It may be intimidating—especially for current or future nurses who are thinking about their commitments to nonviolent respect for the dignity of the human person and God as the Lord of life—to think about the kinds of cases above. But here again is what we hope is a helpful hint: try to think about what would happen if the patient lived. Would those making the decisions here feel like their intention was thwarted? If yes, they were almost certainly aiming at death. If no, they probably were not. Take the example of stopping a child's chemotherapy—would the medical team be upset if after the chemotherapy was stopped the cancer suddenly receded and the child survived? Of course not! And this demonstrates that though they foresee that death is the likely result they are not aiming at death, but rather aiming at something like stopping the child's suffering from the treatment.

On the other hand, we can imagine a scenario where a decision is made to take someone who is "brain-dead" off of a ventilator because the health-care providers thought they no longer had a life worth living and were a burden to the health-care system. In a situation where this patient unexpectedly started breathing it would indeed frustrate the intentions of those making the decision, revealing that they were, in fact, aiming at death. This would of course be a different scenario in which someone says (say in an advanced directive) that they wouldn't want to be "kept alive by machines" and they remove the vent, not because they would be better off dead, but to follow the wish of this patient. In such a case, if the patient started breathing again, they wouldn't be upset. Here they foresaw that death would be the likely result but didn't aim at it. Their goal was simply to take someone off a machine. For those of us who want to focus on choosing to live a certain way, without denying the dignity and goodness of life, these kinds of distinctions become very important.

And we can think in similar ways about abortion of pregnancy—especially in a case where a pregnant woman has cancer of the uterus. Most pro-lifers are OK with the tragic choice a woman may make to remove her uterus even with a baby inside who cannot yet live outside her mother. Suppose (again, to use our little test) there was a mistake made about the baby's gestational age and she survived the hysterectomy—both mother and medical team would be overjoyed and this would reveal that though they foresaw death they were not aiming at it. Unfortunately, most abortions of pregnancy—especially when the baby has an unwanted disability—are clear examples of aiming at death. If an abortion is procured because parents do not want to have a baby with Down syndrome, for instance, the news that their baby has survived the abortion would be most unwelcome and a clear sign that they were aiming at the child's death.

In cases like these we strongly encourage current and future nurses who want to honor their Christian vision of the good to get directly involved in the decision-making processes as essential members of the medical team. Indeed, nurses are often even closer to the decision-making process of the family than are physicians and others on the team, but they are too often left out of the decision-making process overall. The final section of this book will focus on a future for the profession in which nurses have their consciences protected and are welcomed as vital members of the medical team. You deserve the chance to exercise discernment about the above matters for yourself and have your input taken seriously as a co-equal team member.

Before getting to that point, however, we have four more principles and case studies to consider. Next, in chapter 8, we move to examining how a Christian focus on the radical equality of all human beings resists the human-created distinctions based on things like social class and citizenship. We will discuss the implications for how Christian nurses think about their role and their patients.

DISCUSSION QUESTIONS

1. It is worth pointing out that a traditional Christian response to euthanasia and assisted suicide is that killing someone is a violation of human dignity. Maybe groups who support euthanasia and assisted suicide claim to be fighting for death with dignity. How would you

respond to this claim as a Christian nurse? What is going on with the use of the term "dignity" here?

2. This chapter argues that two very similar acts, both of which result in the consequence of death, can be very, very different from a moral perspective. Indeed, one act could be a terrible murder and the other could be a compassionate and moral response to suffering. Does this feel like cheating to you? How might a vision of the good with God as the sole Lord of life help make sense of this position?
3. The role of making patients feel valued when close to death is emphasized in this chapter. What are some examples of how a nurse can make a patient feel valued at the end of life?

8

MATTHEW 25 AND HUMAN-CREATED DISTINCTIONS

The poor need you to draw them out of poverty, and you need the poor to keep you out of Hell.

– Francis Cardinal George
Former Archbishop of Chicago

As suggested by its title, this chapter will focus on the Christian duty to prioritize the ideas and commands Jesus gives us in Matthew 25—and in particular how these ideas and commands resist human-created social distinctions between people. Readers might find themselves surprised by this, at least at first. Haven't we already focused on Matthew 25 in several ways to promote fundamental human equality? What's the point of doing that here again? Asking these questions comes from a good instinct, not least because asking it helps us dig deeper about *what human equality requires* in a culture which—by making human-created social distinctions—treats certain human beings as less than equal.

Unlike previous chapters, this one will focus not on the lack of *fundamental* equality—the kind of inequality which comes from treating certain individuals (like a prenatal child or a "brain-dead" adult) as straight-up nonpersons, or things. Instead, we will focus on the kind of inequality which comes from the preference we give certain human beings based on human-created social distinctions: whether or not one is a citizen, whether or not one is in a prison or other detention facility, or whether or not one is of a certain social class. Those who are marginalized in our culture can still lack basic equality with the rest of us even if no one thinks of them as a non-person. These human-created social distinctions are what lead to the least among us becoming the least among us in the first place. This is especially true in health care in ways that will obviously get our critical attention in this chapter.

REMINDING OURSELVES OF MATTHEW 25

That we have already discussed Matthew 25 in this book should not be a surprise. Especially given that it is concerned with our ultimate destiny after death, there is good reason that it is such a foundational text for so many Christians. Furthermore, one of the primary ways Christ comes to us today is through our encounters with the least among us. As mentioned in chapter 4, our grace-inspired service to the hungry, thirsty, stranger, naked, and imprisoned is not only service to Christ himself, but has an ultimate and eternal impact on our lives. Our grace-inspired decisions about whether and how to relate to the least among us separate out those who will have union with God forever and ever from those who will not. The stakes simply don't get any higher.

The values at the heart of Jesus's commands in Matthew 25—to orient our lives toward serving him in the least among us—run directly counter to the human-created distinctions that have marginalized these populations in the first place. No surprise there. Our Lord commands us to challenge those values that would lead us to treat the stranger from another country differently from someone with the proper papers. Our Lord commands us to directly challenge those values that would lead us to treat the prisoner differently from those who have a spotless criminal record. Our Lord commands us to directly challenge those values which would lead us to treat the poor who cannot afford to eat differently from those with abundance. Indeed, we are commanded to offer them special concern by treating them as we would Christ himself.

This demonstrates, as we have shown throughout this book, just how powerfully counter-cultural an authentic Christian life actually is. It not only resists the kind of consumerism and ableism we've discussed in previous chapters, but it also resists a kind of nationalism that privileges citizens over non-citizens. It resists a kind of classism that privileges those who are "successful" over the "takers" who need social assistance. It even resists the impulse so many of us have to not only ignore but treat with disdain those who have been incarcerated. Jesus does not make distinctions between those who have been rightfully and wrongfully imprisoned. We are commanded to see his holy face in all prisoners. These kinds of dramatically counter-cultural values have radical implications for our whole lives, obviously, but they have particular implications for those in health care and nursing. And it is to these we now turn.

MATTHEW 25 IN NURSING

You will see it in both medicine and nursing, but several kinds of human-created social distinctions have created a hierarchy among the different specialties within health care. There are different perspectives about how to precisely articulate that hierarchy, but it roughly tracks with two factors: (1) how much money one makes and (2) the relative social status of the patients one treats. For instance, orthopedic surgeons working on professional athletes tend to be considered higher than geriatricians caring for nursing home residents. Cardiologists and neurosurgeons are higher than those who practice primary care and family medicine. And so on.

This is probably less pronounced for nurses, although it is still a significant consideration and pressure. A Christian nurse who wishes to follow the commands of Christ in Matthew 25 will run up against a medical culture that, in a very real sense, prioritizes the opposite. If he chooses to focus on caring for the least among us, a nurse will very likely make less money and have less social prestige than if he chose a different, more technical and specialized area of health care. One way to see just how powerful these forces are in medicine is the rising phenomenon of so-called "boutique" medicine aimed at the privileged.[1] Here people of privilege pay directly in cash for their care, and often in the form of a large monthly premium. For example, here are the extra benefits which, according to the website of the "Victors Care" program at the University of Michigan Hospital, patients get if they are able and willing to pay:[2]

- Expertise. "Best-in-class" knowledge from the best physicians UM has to offer.
- No rush. Unhurried visits last as long as the patient deems necessary.
- Direct and extended communication. 24/7 access to talk to one's medical team. Time is provided for "maintaining a dialog and building a relationship for the long term."

Some Christian providers with the UM medical system objected to this program for reasons that should not be difficult to imagine. It puts the most medical resources at the service of the most privileged populations while taking them from those populations on the margins who need them the most. The most talented primary care providers (already in short supply due to the medical culture mentioned above) are poached away from typical practice and put at the service of those who can outbid others for their services. Contrast this preferential treatment with how the economically vulnerable patients are serviced by state Medicaid health insurance. Hospitals and private practices very often lose money when they see such patients due to very low reimbursement rates and thus physicians sometimes feel significant pressure to keep visit length to a minimum. Some refuse to see Medicaid patients altogether.[3] The very things sold to the privileged in "Victors Care" are what the overwhelming majority of economically vulnerable people do not have access to in their health-care coverage.

Now, this is not to say all private practices or clinics that are cash-pay are bad. Far from it. Alisha has personally seen benefits to patients from these types of clinics. As a health-care provider herself, she fully supports providers stepping outside of the traditional models of care for Matthew 25–centered reasons. It is uncommon to see private practices nowadays, as most have been closed down or bought out by larger health-care systems.[4] In these larger organizations, providers have much less say in how the clinic is run. Appointment times are limited and the focus has shifted to productivity pay, meaning there is a push to see a higher number of patients each day and to perform more procedures. And the restrictions that insurance put on providers can make it even more of a challenge. For many providers, these obstacles are a large part of burnout. More providers are looking to leave the traditional model and provide care the way they feel best meets the patients' needs, especially economically vulnerable patients who, because they are often sicker, need more of the provider's time for less cost per visit. The problem comes when the market rears its ugly head and medicine serves the rich and privileged at the expense of the poor and marginalized.

Those of us claimed by Christ, however, must explicitly reject this way of thinking about health care. Abandoning the least among us, given that it means abandoning Christ himself, imperils our very salvation. Growing up and living in the Westernized culture we do can make this difficult, no question. But if we take the fullness of Matthew 25 seriously, it becomes even worse than this. Think, for instance, about the dramatic disadvantages those who have been incarcerated face. Even common diseases like influenza hit these particular populations hard; the COVID-19 pandemic was an absolute disaster in US jails and prisons.[5] But as difficult as it may be for our culture to hear, the incarcerated population bears the face of Christ and deserves preferential treatment. Abandoning them in favor of those with more privilege puts us at risk of eternal separation from God: so reads the clear warning of Matthew 25. Happily, a significant number of Christians in health care are making good on this obligation.[6]

Another concerning trend is the rising number of patients who live in Health Professional Shortage Areas (HPSA). Nearly eighty million people live in areas where there are health-care shortages—meaning no access to prevention screenings, basic care, or immunizations. Most of these places are rural. Primary care remains the biggest shortage in rural areas. However, advanced practice nurses (midwives and nurse practitioners) are answering the call. They are more likely to move to these areas to provide primary care to the patients in need.[7] And many do it not as an advantageous career move, but as a calling.

When one lives and works in an idolatrous culture that puts the good of the secular nation-state ahead of the commands of Jesus and vision of the gospel, it can be particularly difficult to live out the part of Matthew 25 which asks us to see the Lord's face in the stranger. This is especially true given that Christ makes no distinction between caring for strangers who are legal citizens of the culture and those who do not have their proper papers. Tragically, however, many cultures use human-created categories to make precisely these kinds of distinctions, including ones that deny whole classes of people access to basic health care. Facing even more obstacles than do Medicaid patients, undocumented immigrants have been denied access to COVID-19 vaccines—despite being disproportionately represented in the dangerous jobs of frontline workers (especially in meatpacking and other food preparation), which put them at particular risk for contracting the virus.[8] It is counter-cultural, but even here the Christian health-care provider must put aside human-created nationalistic distinctions in favor of the clear requirements of the gospel. And the clear requirement of the gospel is to see the face of Christ in strangers.[9]

CASE STUDY: THE IRWIN DETENTION CENTER

Perhaps more often than we'd like to admit, multiple categories of vulnerability that Christ mentions in Matthew 25 apply to the same group of people, making them even *more* vulnerable. Such is the case for undocumented immigrants detained by the United States. One example of this extreme vulnerability took place in Irwin Detention Center (IDC) in Georgia and made national headlines in September 2020. Owned by a private prison company named LaSalle Corrections, IDC's practices were made public by a whistleblower nurse named Dawn Wooten. Based at first on her testimony alone and later on the testimony of the residents themselves, we learned of "jarring medical neglect" at IDC. This included refusing "to test detained immigrants for COVID-19 who have been exposed to the virus and are symptomatic" and "allowing employees to work while they are symptomatic awaiting COVID-19 test results." The cover-up of their actions included "shredding of medical requests submitted by detained immigrants" and "fabricating medical records."[10]

"You don't want to see what you're seeing," Wooten told *The Intercept* in one of a series of interviews. Her resistance to IDC's practices began when she was told to triage the first detainee who tested positive for COVID-19. Having no mask, she refused to do so. As her complaints ramped up, administrators retaliated by dropping her hours before demoting her to being fully on-call and only scheduling a few hours of work a month for her. Little mattered to IDC other than profit: "They keep piling more people in here. They keep bringing more people in here, and in the end, it's all about the money," said a detained woman who had to wait over a week for her sick call. Wooten agreed: "They get seen as a dollar sign. Their heads are counted not as humans but as dollars."[11]

And the situation worsened. Wooten expressed frustration and anger at the number of detained immigrant women at IDC who received hysterectomies. While the procedure was likely medically indicated for some women, she noted ominously that "everybody's uterus cannot be that bad." And she went on to explain in more detail:

> Everybody he sees has a hysterectomy—just about everybody. He's even taken out the wrong ovary on a young lady [detained immigrant woman]. She was supposed to get her left ovary removed because it had a cyst on the left ovary; he took out the right one. She was upset. She had to go back to take out the left and she wound up with a total hysterectomy. She still wanted children—so she has to go back home now and tell her husband that she can't bear kids . . . she said she was not all the way out under anesthesia and heard him [doctor] tell the nurse that he took the wrong ovary.[12]

There seems to have been one physician—who Wooten said was dubbed "the uterus collector" by detainees—who was particularly awful in his treatment of patients. The *New York Times* interviewed sixteen women who were concerned about the gynecological treatment they received at the IDC and compiled a major investigative report.They had four independent, board-certified gynecologists associated with medical schools review the patients' medical records and all found that Dr. Amin ("the uterus collector") "seemed to consistently recommend surgical intervention, even when it did not seem medically necessary at the time and nonsurgical treatment options were available."[13]

Indeed, one of his patients, an undocumented immigrant named Wendy Dowe who had been in detention for four months after living for two decades in the United States, said that Amin told her that her uterus had large cysts and masses that needed to be removed. She was skeptical, but Amin insisted "and as a detainee—brought to the hospital in handcuffs and shackles—she felt pressured to consent." She didn't learn the truth until after she was deported to Jamaica; doctors there saw that the cysts were small, normal, and did not require surgical intervention. In another case, a thirty-six-year-old immigrant from Mexico asked to be seen after experiencing pain in her ribs stemming from physical abuse by an ex-partner. "I was assuming they were going to check my rib," she said. "The next thing I know, he's doing a vaginal exam." Dr. Amin put in his notes that she had complained of heavy menstruation and pelvic pain even though she had done no such thing. The end result was this patient undergoing a major surgical gynecological procedure that she had not expected. "I woke up and I was alone, and I was in pain and everyone spoke English so I could not ask any questions," she said. The *Times* notes that three days later she was deported.[14]

This story "bears striking similarities" to others the *Times*'s panel of physicians reviewed. The reporter of the story correctly and provocatively notes that independent doctors like Amin are paid for the procedures they perform with Department of Homeland Security funds. Procedures like the ones just described are billed at thousands of dollars each, a lucrative prospect. This is not the first time Amin has been under this kind of scrutiny. In 2013 he was named with several other doctors in a civil case claiming that they had over-billed Medicare and Medicaid.[15] But the financial incentive is only part of the story here. The incredibly vulnerable situation of an immigrant population in shackles and cuffs who do not speak the language of their health-care providers is at least as important. Incredibly, they were made even more vulnerable by speaking with the *Times* and *Intercept*. A class-action lawsuit filed five months after these stories came out alleges "women and others held at the facility were placed in solitary confinement, experienced physical assault and were deported—or nearly deported—for speaking up about Amin."[16] Only a federal lawsuit stopped four crucial witnesses for both the civil suit and an ongoing federal investigation from being deported.

CASE ANALYSIS

On one level, analysis of this case should not be all that complex. If the testimony of Wooten and the detainees is accurate, then what has occurred here is an unconscionable breach of fundamental medical ethics agreed upon by virtually everyone. Providers were apparently either incredibly sloppy with informed consent or ignored it altogether. And they did so with multiple surgical procedures that had the potential to affect perhaps the most important and personal aspect of someone's life: their procreative and reproductive capability. Upon learning of this case, we found it difficult not to hear the echoes of racist eugenic practices in the past, particularly given our previous discussion of this ideology in the US and Nazi Germany in the first part of the twentieth century. Is it possible that Dr. Amin and colleagues who at least looked the other way in the IDC did not make value judgments about what kind of people should be having children?

Even if this wasn't the entirety of what was going on, this case also highlights a theme we have established throughout this book: the difference between (1) Christ-centered health care focused on care for a real, live person in front of the provider and (2) the technocratic practices of health-care providers who focus more on procedures rather than on the holistic good of their patients. As we have demonstrated, contemporary hospitals have lost their original Christian meaning of care and hospitality and are now primarily places of technical intervention against a patient's particular disease. And the good here is nothing to denigrate—thank God we can intervene to save and improve lives in the ways this technology now permits. Some people reading this book right now are only able to do so because of such developments in medicine.

But we also saw that there is a darker side to this trend toward medical technocracy: with the way the US health-care system is now, most health-care providers now derive their authority, money, and social standing primarily from their technical training and expertise. Caring for their patients in the fullness of who they are is a secondary consideration—especially when building relationships over (unpaid) time is necessary to do it. If Dr. Amin, a specialist physician who focused on doing lucrative procedures, had instead prioritized the holistic good of the person in front of him, he would never have been capable of committing such terrible acts. The physicians who reviewed the medical notes for the case agreed that his actions did not line up with ethical treatment. Let's remember it was a nurse, Wooten, who ended up blowing the whistle. She put a version of this point beautifully during a press conference: "As a nurse, I took an oath that my life, when I step in, no longer was my life; it became the lives of others. And until you see through the eyes of others and you experience through the eyes of others, there's no concern, and there's no regard."[17] So there's a level on which virtually anyone with a conscience can see what is wrong in this case. But there's a deeper level on which we can and should focus our theological moral analysis as well. What are we to make of the "jarring medical neglect" this undocumented population experiences? What are we to make of the lack of concern for COVID-19 infections? And, even outside of a detention context, what are we to make of a refusal to treat these patients as we would other frontline workers when it came to vaccine distribution?

It doesn't take too much to imagine how many react, given the human-created distinctions that dominate our culture. "Aren't these people law-breakers? Don't they take resources away from actual citizens? What about immigrants who followed the rules and waited in line? What about those who are currently waiting to enter the country? How is it fair that these illegal immigrants get treated the same as those who follow the rules?" For many embedded in the current American culture, this seems something like common sense. But this, once again, shows just how little influence the gospel has on the way our culture forms its citizens. This disparity is nothing new: Christ's practices in this area were counter-cultural in his time as well. Remember how often he was criticized by those who had power and prestige (particularly the scribes, Pharisees, and scholars of the law) for the kind of company he kept and the people on whom he focused? Tax collectors, prostitutes, gentiles, and more. One particularly poignant example, from Luke 7:36–50, was when a "sinful woman" anointed him with her ointment and the Pharisee hosting him doubted whether Jesus could be a prophet if he didn't know that the woman was a sinner. The unspoken assumption behind his words was that *of course* a holy person wouldn't associate with such a person, much less given her priority for his ministry. In health care, do we also wrestle with this same concern?

There have been so many situations over the course of my (Alisha) career as both a nurse and a nurse practitioner where a patient's social status, criminal history, or financial status impacted the care they received. I am sure there were times where I prejudged a patient before ever hearing their full story. There were times when a prisoner would come to the floor with a police escort. I met parents accused of child abuse when I cared for their children. I worked in a homeless shelter, caring for patients struggling with drug addiction, severe mental illness, and many other tragic situations. What changed my heart the most toward some of these patients was hearing their stories and remembering they were fundamentally hurting people in need of care. Some had such terrible pasts; anyone hearing the story would be tearful. There was one patient I met who opened my eyes the most to how much bigger my role was as a nurse. He was a new patient and was there to establish care. When I walked into the room he quickly got up and showed me his ID card and said by law he needed to let me know that he was just released from prison and was staying at a halfway house. He appeared very nervous, but pleasant. I felt God moving me during this appointment. I asked the patient how long he had been in prison. His reply shocked me . . . over thirty years! I asked him if he was open to sharing his story with me. He was in prison for murder. If I had let him stop his story there, I would have missed a wonderful opportunity. I questioned him a bit more and he went on to tell me about his life. He grew up in a home where he witnessed drug abuse regularly. His grandmother ran a prostitution ring out of the home. All he ever witnessed were drugs, violence, and darkness. He had no real education. He experienced nothing but tragedy. He was now trying to navigate a whole new world as a free man. I saw him several times over the next few months. I could see hope grow in him about his future and he talked a lot about God. One day I walked into his room and he had tears in his eyes. I asked if he was okay, and after a few moments of silence he stated, "You are the first nice person I have met in my life." He was nearly sixty years old and it took that long for someone to show him kindness. Sure, I helped him with his new adult-onset diabetes and got his blood pressure under control. But what this patient needed, and what every patient needs, was kindness, compassion, and the assurance that they matter and are loved. I am so thankful he walked into my life to remind me of that. We see this enacted in how Jesus responded to the sinful woman. He turned conventional social wisdom (based on human-created distinctions) on its head with the way he treated this woman, even claiming that her faith was greater than that of the Pharisee hosting the gathering.

We are called to imitate our Lord's example here—even when it doesn't seem fair or just by human standards. Remember the parable of the generous vineyard owner in Matthew 20:1–18? He hired various workers at different times of day, from nine in the morning until five in the late afternoon, but when it came time to be paid all the workers received the same wage, including those who had worked only one hour. When those who were hired in the morning grumbled that they had been treated unfairly, the owner reminded them that he paid them the agreed-upon amount and they should not be envious because he had been generous with the other workers. This, then, is the image Jesus offers us of the generous, overflowing, merciful love of God. Love which *is* God. The love that, according to the commandment Christ tells us is the greatest, we are to prioritize above everything else in our life. And the second-greatest commandment insists that we must treat our neighbor with this love as well.

And who is our neighbor? Christ, as we've seen earlier in this book, answers that question by telling the Parable of the Good Samaritan, a parable that highlights the refusal of a foreigner (unlike the "better" classes of people as the hearer would have understood them) to cross to the other side of the road when he was confronted with a stranger in need of medical attention. Moved with the generous, overflowing, and merciful love of God, the Good Samaritan immediately stops what he is doing, puts his own plans on hold, loads the injured man on his own animal, and walks to the nearest inn where he can purchase a room for him and pay for his care. He also insists on coming back to check on him, committing to an extended relationship with a total stranger. This is a love that is beyond reason and beyond human-created distinctions of national citizenship and social class. It is also the kind of love about which Christ commands us, "Go and do likewise."

For nurses like Dawn Wooten, this kind of love is very much consistent with the way she understands her vocation and what is required at the place she has chosen to work. This love was something that gave her life energy, direction, and profound meaning. It motivated her to courageously resist and call out the injustices her patients were facing, even when she faced severe consequences. It is also the case, however, that the kind of place she has chosen to work was quite low on the social hierarchy of medical prestige. But as we will explore in the next chapter, this is precisely where Christians are called to be.

DISCUSSION QUESTIONS

1. This chapter says that human-created distinctions have erected a hierarchy among the different specialties in health care. What do these distinctions reveal about what we value in persons? What drives these value judgments and how does your Christian faith flip this value system on its head, so to speak?
2. Jesus's command in Matthew 25:40—to orient our lives toward serving him in the least among us—runs counter to the culture today. How can Christian nurses follow this command when caring for patients?
3. One of the most important human-created distinctions discussed today is between citizens and noncitizens of a nation-state. Noncitizen strangers bear the face of Christ in a special way. What claims does that fact make on a Christian?

9

THE LAST SHALL BE FIRST

> Even the weakest and most vulnerable, the sick, the old, the unborn, and the poor, are masterpieces of God's creation, made in his own image, destined to live forever, and deserving of the utmost reverence and respect.
>
> – *Pope Francis*

For those of us raised in a culture that prioritizes getting ahead—especially if we do not have the strength of someone like Dawn Wooten, the fearless nurse we learned about in the previous chapter—it can be a daunting task to live out the Christian idea of "the last shall be first." The last shall be first means turning conventional wisdom on its head, putting aside our selfish interests as understood by the world, and living an *incredibly* counter-cultural life. As we mentioned in chapters 2 and 4, it means following the example of the Sisters of Mercy who knew, taught, and lived out the truth that authentic power comes not from domination, but rather from service to others. You want power? Die to self and embrace your weakness. You want glory? Embrace humility and even humiliation. You want to be first? Put others before you. The Sisters of Mercy knew that any authentic power they held came from putting the love of the marginalized ahead of their personal interests.

So the last shall be first not only means putting the most vulnerable first (as we discussed in the previous chapter); for Christians it also means we should be open to God's call to service and ministry, which the surrounding culture considers "last." We must do this even if we feel intense social pressure to put our worldly, selfish interests first. We are called to resist the sin of pride and to humble ourselves in the service of others. A desire for prestige, for a certain kind of lifestyle, and using one's patients as a means to an end puts us at terrible risk for undermining the central message of the gospel of Jesus Christ.

NURSING CARE UNDERSTOOD AS PUTTING ASIDE ONE'S SELFISH DESIRES

Though nurses are by no means immune from the social expectations of the world and temptations toward pride, the very nature of nursing as a profession helps to resist such temptations. An intense focus on caring for the reality of individual patients in front of them and also for families and communities tends to take the focus off of oneself and shift it onto one's vocation or calling as a giver of care. A giver of care to patients who, rather than merely a collection of organs that need treatment and maintenance, are persons with a holistic reality that calls us out of ourselves and into their reality. As we will see particularly in the next chapter, because nurses care for patients who are always in relationship with others, this is also true for whole communities. Good Christian nurses put their patients and the communities in which they live before their own selfish desires.

From our discussion in the previous chapter, it should now be clear that nurses inevitably come across vulnerable patients: the elderly, children, the unborn, patients with disabilities, patients addicted to drugs, homeless patients, immigrants, and those suffering from mental illness. And we know that for a variety of reasons, certain populations are more vulnerable to sickness and disease: the elderly, people of color, the poor, and so on. These patients are typically the ones who have limited access to health care as well. We have already discussed how care for the sick on the margins of society has been a profound ministry of the church for centuries. The shift to practicing medicine as a money-making enterprise (which is closely connected to how medicine now assigns prestige) has made this much more difficult—especially given that those who need care the most often have the least ability to pay to receive even the least amount of care.

We believe that basic health care is a fundamental right for human beings, something necessary for basic human flourishing, and it is a good that those who need it can demand from others. Their need produces a duty on our part. Significantly, this is a truth articulated by Scripture, Roman Catholic teaching, and even the World Health Organization—an organization which highlighted this in their constitution nearly seventy years ago: "The enjoyment of the highest attainable standard of health is one of the fundamental rights of every human being without distinction of race, religion, political belief, economic or social condition."[1] Unfortunately, we have a long way to go to reach this goal. In part, this is because we do not see the claims of the most vulnerable as trumping our selfish desires.

Nurses see health inequities demanding our attention in many different places: whether it is in acute care settings, home health care, nursing homes, or public health. We've shared a few of these examples already, such as the previous chapter's example of the undocumented immigrant patient who was denied health care. Other examples include nursing home patients who are over medicated and sedated so that health-care workers don't have to spend time and resources on them. We see nonverbal patients who lie in their beds, neglected, developing untreated pressure ulcers. We see an astonishing amount of untreated mental illness, especially in the homeless population.

We also see these kinds of inequities on a much broader scale. Large numbers of patients living in rural areas often have little to no access to basic care. Patients living in lower socioeconomic areas are often affected by environmental hazards that make them more vulnerable to disease at the same time they have limited access to quality care. And then there's the large number of patients who are simply turned away (or never show up for an appointment in the first place) because they lack the ability to pay. Nurses who put selfish desires aside in choosing to care for these populations should expect to be regularly and personally confronted with the injustices our most vulnerable face. But armed with a holistic model of nursing care, their response to the just demands of the least ones puts them in a position to be local, national, and international leaders in caring for these populations. There are organizations and groups who are doing just that. Certain charities like Samaritan's Purse, Physicians for Human Rights, Doctors Without Borders, and free health clinics, which are often run by volunteer staff, are dedicated toward caring for the underserved.

Dr. Dennis Sansom's moral examination of the opportunity Christian nurses have in making good on their duty to put the least in the most prominent place is of particular interest:

> If society understands itself as a community bound together by an overriding moral purpose, as did Israel and the early church and as Aristotle described the natural law of all cities/states, then each citizen must contribute to that purpose, and the community must provide ways in which each citizen can participate in that moral purpose. Therefore, the church should find ways not only to promote healthcare for the poor but to identify with the poor through such means as providing clinics and hospices for those left out of healthcare networks, joining hospitals and clinics with a ministerial presence, giving aesthetic ways to witness to the sick and poor Christ's redemptive work, and ordaining healthcare workers to serve as ministers in their medical work.[2]

And while nurses are generally very good at putting their patients ahead of selfish desires, it is still a profession that can fall prey to believing the world's ideas about (and measuring scale for) what is valuable. We mentioned in the previous chapter, for instance, that geriatrics—although one of the best fields for a nurse with Christian values—is low on the health-care hierarchy of power and prestige. Some of this is related to the ableism and ageism we've discussed in previous chapters. Some of this is related to the relative lack of money made in this field compared to other fields. And this is a bias that infiltrates many professions within health care, including, unfortunately, nursing. There is a serious nursing shortage overall in the United States, but it is particularly pronounced in nursing homes where residents often suffer terrible neglect due to the lack of available nurses. Indeed, the COVID-19 pandemic hit the world over the head with the reality of a terrible lack of care in nursing homes, due in part to a lack of caregivers.[3] This problem was particularly heartbreaking for those with dementia.[4]

For the central case study of this chapter, we highlight the story of an elderly and vulnerable patient who the health-care system not only failed to protect, but who also had her basic dignity violated in grossly inappropriate ways.

THE ELDERLY AND DISABLED: A CASE OF PROFOUND NEGLECT

Elder abuse and neglect have become growing and urgent problems. Diabolically, patients with dementia (some of the most vulnerable patients in all of health care) are at higher risk than neurotypical elderly patients. The numbers are just terrible: nearly half of patients with dementia have experienced abuse or neglect.[5] We want to invite readers to give full attention to the specific story we tell below, but we should underscore that what follows is anything but an isolated example.

Between 2007 and 2008, a ninety-year-old Massachusetts resident by the name of Genevieve was living in a nursing home.

Genevieve suffered from dementia.[6] After seven months of care, she fell out of her wheelchair onto the floor. She was admitted to the hospital, at which point her medical team found that she was suffering from several complications: an untreated pressure ulcer on her back, a severe urinary tract infection, sepsis, uncontrolled blood sugars, dehydration, and renal failure, among other acute problems. Most of these complications could have been avoided if she had received even the most basic medical care at her nursing home. Unfortunately, none of the problems were being treated by the staff who were supposed to care for her.[7] While the hospital attempted to treat these conditions, her symptoms were too far advanced by the time she arrived. Genevieve passed away in August 2008.

During her stay at the nursing home, Genevieve complained of symptoms before her fall. Her family brought up these concerns to the nursing home staff who repeatedly assured the family that Genevieve was doing well. Upon further questioning, they were told that she was merely experiencing a flu that was circulating around the facility.[8] It took Genevieve's fall out of the wheelchair to get her to the hospital where her real medical issues were uncovered.

Genevieve's family opened a lawsuit against the nursing home. According to the lawsuit, an investigation revealed the nursing home failed to hire competent staff and did not provide proper training. The complaint also stated that the owners of the nursing home required staff to recruit heavier care residents to the facility—which meant higher reimbursement—despite the fact that the current residents' needs exceeded the capacity of the staff.[9] There were also issues with charting. In one example, Genevieve's chart was marked that she was turned in bed—a basic practice to help prevent pressure ulcers—when in fact she was not even in the facility on the days it was charted. The jury found the nursing home was at fault and awarded the family $14.5 million in the wrongful death and negligence case.[10]

WHY WAS GENEVIEVE NEGLECTED TO DEATH?

In some ways, this case is the paradigmatic example of what happens when the Christian principle of "the last shall be first" is completely ignored and even actively resisted by the surrounding culture. Elderly people with dementia should be among the *most* prioritized populations in health care, but Genevieve's case reveals some important reasons why something close to the opposite is true. Even when there is enough staffing in a nursing home, nurses and nursing aides are often not properly trained and sometimes even grossly incompetent. This stems in large measure from the fact that it is difficult to recruit nurses and physicians to work in these homes. And this stems in large measure from the fact that there is comparatively little money and prestige (by the world's standards) to be gained from working in this area of health care. Thus, nursing homes are often forced either to hire fewer staff than they need or hire staff who are not willing or competent to treat these patients with the care they are owed.

There is pervasive ageism in our culture, which works hand in glove with our culture's worship of youth. And, in a related way, ageism works with our worship of "independence" and "autonomy." These are illusions, of course, and the next chapter will focus on how humans are always in relationships on which we depend: with God, with our families, and with local and distant communities. Much of the time, however, the surrounding culture can set up effective illusions which, appealing to our sense of pride, can falsely convince us that we are fully independent and autonomous beings. But the very existence of the elderly provides an incisive reminder about just how frail and dependent human life actually is. It directly dispels the illusions the surrounding culture needs to keep these myths alive. Christian nurses, however, go into their profession already disabused of this notion. We are firmly aware of our reliance on God and neighbor. All life is a gift. It is the vice of pride that tempts us to believe the illusions of independence and autonomy. Thus, Christian nurses who care for the elderly are not threatened or turned away by the dramatic ways in which this population relies upon others. Instead, they see fellow dependent and finite human beings whose needs are only more visible than their own, not different in kind. Every single one of us is a totally dependent and contingent creature.

There is also an aspect of dementia that we believe ought to be highlighted here. Based in part on discussions we've had in previous chapters about fundamental human equality, we already know that the move to a "Trait X" vision of equality has left out many kinds of human beings. To prenatal children and individuals with catastrophic brain injuries, we may need to add human beings with dementia as the next population to fail to count as "full persons" (therefore having fundamental and social equality with other human beings). If, for instance, "Trait X" is rationality or self-awareness, then it is just a fact that many people with later-stage dementia have lost these traits. Many others with even milder forms of the disease have their capacity for rationality and self-awareness quite diminished.

The secular philosopher Peter Singer at Princeton has been arguing for decades about what it has meant that the surrounding culture has rejected a Christian ethic of fundamental human equality. We *strongly* disagree with his views, yet we also have a grudging respect for his consistency and push for conclusions that follow from the culture's values, but have yet to be fully implemented. He has argued, for instance, that if one is pro-choice for abortion, then one should also be pro-choice for infanticide—given that neither prenatal children nor neonatal children are rational or self-aware beings. He has also argued that if one argues human beings who are "brain-dead" or in a (so-called) persistent vegetative state do not count the same as the rest of us because they are not rational or self-aware, then the same is true of people with late-stage dementia.

Eventually this point of view would be one he'd confront in his own life when his mother, Cora Singer, developed dementia. Though he ended up providing care for her, he never gave up on the argument he was making, only saying, "Perhaps it is more difficult than I thought before, because it is different when it's your mother."[11] Can the consistent neglect of people with dementia be totally disconnected from the culture's claim that what matters about "us" is that we are rational, self-aware, autonomous, and independent? We think not. This is why we believe it is so very important for a Christian understanding of fundamental human equality to be vigorously defended in our culture.[12]

GOING INTO GERIATRIC CARE?

Just as the church has many parts in one body (1 Cor. 12:12–27), so too does health care. Though Christian nurses do have specific values and obligations they must bring to their vocation, it of course does not follow that everyone should do the same thing. We are all called by God to play different roles and parts in the functioning of the whole. That said, especially in light of what we have presented in this chapter, we want to strongly encourage Christian nurses to consider working in geriatrics. Disabled elderly populations bear the holy face of Christ in a special way, but what makes this area of health care different is the intense need that it is facing—both now and in the future.

We already lack the resources to give these populations the care they deserve, but especially as those who make it to older ages tend to live longer and longer, the problem will go from bad to horrific if nothing changes. If the rate of increase is the same over the next three decades, the Harvard NeuroDiscovery Center estimates that in the US alone *twelve million more people* will have neurodegenerative diseases. Worldwide, more than fifty million people are living with dementia; that number is projected to double every twenty years.[13] Addressing this mammoth problem is going to take a fundamental shift in how we think about what kinds of health-care careers to pursue, and how nurses can be leaders in transforming health care for this population. Christians can and should lead the way in resisting the current cultural incentives to neglect the basic needs of these populations. If we fail to act, if we fail to change how we think about geriatrics, we see only one of two options available to us: (1) massive euthanasia by passive neglect and/or active injections, or (2) a slouch toward more depersonalization of this population by having them cared for by robots.[14] Both are terrible options from the standpoint of preserving human dignity.

While most nursing work is difficult, geriatrics can be particularly difficult. Moving patients to avoid bedsores; changing their clothes and diapers and bedpans; trying to calm, console, and feed those who are angry or otherwise distressed: these are all very difficult parts of the job. Other aspects of nursing may seem easier and therefore perhaps more appealing, particularly if it makes one more money. But the other side of the story here is that being Christ for these patients—and seeing Christ in them—is one of the most rewarding and fulfilling things that Christian nurses who have worked in geriatrics have ever experienced.

Alisha has experienced this firsthand. Indeed, her first experience in health care was in a nursing home. She spent two years as a nursing assistant during her teenage years. This was a pivotal time in her life as both a Christian and as a young woman trying to figure out her calling. She believes this experience—being given the incredible responsibility of caring for patients at one of their most vulnerable stages in life—shaped her entire path. The act of washing someone's feet, literally, can change a heart. In the years since that time, Alisha has worked with many patients in their later years and discovered that there is no generation more grateful for care and compassion than this population of patients. One of the reasons the elderly are often dismissed by health-care providers or their care is subpar is, frankly, that nurses and physicians see the elderly as somehow less human. Not as someone's father or mother or sister or brother. They are maybe even looked at as a drain on the system or judged by their perceived low quality of life. But when we care for someone—truly care for someone—we don't look for what we get in return. We comfort them in need, we talk to them with love and respect, we put ourselves in their shoes and love them where they are, and sometimes we wash their feet.

Charlie has a friend he's calling "Annella" (to protect her anonymity) who worked during her nursing training as a certified nursing assistant in a nursing home during the pandemic. She told him many stories about neglect and death (including terrible examples of her patients being dehydrated and abandoned to death), but also stories of the triumph of human dignity that she was able to foster as part of her care for this population. Here's one particularly moving story she told:

> I think "Rebecca" was one of my favorites. The first time I met her, she was on the fourth floor, rehab, and she had just come back from the hospital. The fourth floor was packed. Everyone was coming in from the hospital, and everyone was on droplet precautions so that meant we had to gown and mask up before even entering their rooms—only there weren't enough gowns and we only had one mask for a week. Lights were going off constantly and there was only one other CNA with me. We did nothing but run all night.
>
> The rehab floor isn't for residents. There's nothing homey about it, it's more like a hotel, except with ports for tubes coming out of the walls, and hospital beds and bathrooms. It's one, long hallway, and Rebecca was in the second to last room.
>
> She had been a local photographer, a professional, and she was beautiful. You could tell that she used to carry herself gracefully. But when I met her, she was in a hospital gown

> with an IV attached to her and she had soaked through the diaper, her pressure injury wound pad was saturated along with the bed, and she was crying.
>
> I don't know how long she'd been left there by herself, but it had been a long time. The look on her face was of lost hope. I think that was the first time I got really angry at the injustice of all of it.
>
> Changing patients is like a choreographed dance. You gather your supplies, you put the bed up high, and you do everything in halves—you strip half of the bed, roll them away from you, tuck everything tight under them, roll them back to you, and the same with the diapers. Roll, roll, roll. It takes so much out of them, when they have so little energy to spare that it's exhausting. But I got her cleaned up, dry, we washed her face, put cream on her arms and legs, got fresh sheets on, and I got her covered up with fresh sheets and a blanket. Pretty soon Rebecca was as snug as a bug in a rug, fast asleep with a very different look on her face.

Annella will soon finish her nursing degree and, despite all the struggles of the pandemic, has decided to continue to serve the geriatric population as a registered nurse. She is that fulfilled by the work.

THE JOY OF LIVING THE GOSPEL

Many outside the nursing profession find this kind of fulfillment in working with aging adults as well. Erin Youkins is currently the Respect Life Coordinator for the Archdiocese of Baltimore, but before that she worked with the elderly in nursing home and occupational therapy contexts. We asked if she could share something about this experience. Here was her reply; you will notice an overlap with Alisha's experiences:

> Working with aging adults throughout my career has been an unexpected gift to me and has, without a doubt, brought me closer to God. The generosity of spirit from so many of my patients, the desire to encourage, to share their wisdom and experience, and the genuine gratitude they often expressed, was more than inspirational to me—it was transformative. Even when illness had robbed a patient of their thoughts, memory, or ability to speak, a relationship was possible and the opportunity to dignify someone in need was a chance for me to serve Jesus. I have no doubt that every beating heart has great value and is deserving of great care until it is called home by God. Encountering Christ in the people I was blessed to serve, and the opportunity to do some good for others, was often times much more therapeutic to my own soul than any therapy I could provide for them.

This is the kind of joy and fulfillment that comes to people who live the gospel, even if they appear to be toiling or suffering from the perspective of the world. This is how it can be true that we are called to the cross while still making sense of Jesus saying that his yoke is easy and his burden light. A Christian (bio)ethic turns the conventional wisdom of the world on its head. If one chooses to engage with the elderly population, then one may not be wealthy or enjoy the prestige that comes from other kinds of health care. But who is richer than someone who has this kind of happiness and joy? Who has more authentic prestige than someone who is so deeply fulfilled by their work?

That these kinds of relationships are so life-giving should not surprise Christians who know that these are the kinds of creatures God made us to be. We are made to be in a relationship of service to others. Indeed, our very identity cannot be separated from our relationships with others. This, of course, has profound implications for what it means for a nurse to act on behalf of her patients. And that is the subject of the next chapter.

DISCUSSION QUESTIONS

1. The authors of this chapter claim that basic health care is a fundamental right for human beings. Do you agree with this? How might you respond to those who think differently?
2. Recall the following quote from the chapter: "Being Christ for [geriatric patients]—and seeing Christ in them—is one of the most rewarding and fulfilling things that Christian nurses who have worked in geriatrics have ever experienced." This model of care should be the model not only in geriatrics, but in all patient populations. What does it mean for you to be Christ to your patients in different kinds of health-care settings?
3. Right now the health-care systems in most Western countries have a bias against the elderly and disabled. What specific things do you feel need to happen in order to improve care for these, some of the most vulnerable populations we have?

10

NEVER NOT IN RELATIONSHIP

> Our relationship with each other is the criterion the world uses to judge whether our message is truthful–Christian community is the final apologetic.
>
> – *Francis Schaeffer*

If someone said, "Tell me about yourself," how would you answer the question? Almost certainly you would make reference to explicit or implicit relationships. Your being part of a family, for instance: someone's son or daughter, brother or sister, aunt or uncle, and so on. Or you might discuss being a nursing student at a particular school or an employee at a certain hospital or clinic. Or being a part of real or virtual community associated with a sport, hobby, or other mutual interest you have. If you are reading this book, you would likely discuss your church and, of course, the most important relationship you have of all: the one you have with your Creator. If you were to mention your favorite music or movies, you invoke an implicit connection with the people who created them. Indeed, the very fact you would be using language (likely English) to answer this question means you are by definition participating in a complex relationship of symbols and shared meaning within a set of relationships and communities. There is no escaping our essential nature as relational creatures. This is simply what it means to be human.

And this, of course, is the way we have been created. As we discussed in chapter 4, God made us in the image and likeness of himself: a triune God whose very essence is to be in relationship. This One-God-Who-Is-Trinity entered into our own human reality through the person of Jesus Christ through the Holy Spirit, thus making us all brothers and sisters through his incarnation. We are deeply and profoundly related to each other in ways that, while not erasing our differences, unite us in the very essence of who we are. Saint Paul reminds us that we are all one in Christ Jesus (Gal. 3:28). Chapter 4 also emphasized that this Christian vision resists our culture's tendency toward individualism. Too often we see our relationships with others as a burden to our individual freedom and autonomy. But this image of the radically autonomous free agent, one who is able to exert an individual will without the limitations of given relationships with (and obligations to) others, is not consistent with a Christian vision of the inherent relationality at the heart of human nature.

Recall from chapter 9 and elsewhere throughout the book how an undue focus on the individual (and especially the supposedly *autonomous* individual) works to marginalize vulnerable populations who are most visibly dependent on others. This false individualism gives rise to the kind of persistent ableism and ageism that, as we have discussed, plagues contemporary medicine and our broader culture. In this chapter, we will wrestle more deeply with the false and dangerous vision of human patients as isolated individuals making autonomous decisions. Human beings are never not in mutually dependent relationships with others. Human beings can only be fully ourselves in relationships with others, especially our families and those with whom we have genuine, embodied relationships.

NURSING AS CARE FOR PEOPLE IN RELATIONSHIPS

In some ways, the profession of nursing itself is a paradigmatic example of living out the truth of a Christian vision of the human being in relationship. As we mentioned in the previous chapter, nurses care for actual people in the fullness of their human reality. The fullness of the reality of their patients summons nurses out of themselves and into a relationship with their (often very vulnerable) patients. And because nurses learn more about the relationships many patients bring into their moment of illness and vulnerability, they can bring this knowledge to the health-care team who may be more focused on a specific system or problem.

Nurses, for instance, are most often the ones consistently interacting with the father, the sister, the best friend, the spouse, or the partner of the patient. Indeed, nurses are often the ones most aware of just how deeply involved families are in the care and decision-making processes of patients. It should be stated, though, that with the rise in fragmented care the continuity of care is being threatened, leading to the compromise of nurse-patient relationships. When this happens, nurses are not able to spend the time with patients to gain an understanding of who they are—especially in the context of the patient's relationships—and what their greatest needs are. In the United States, "individual patient autonomy" is often held in the highest regard such that we imagine that the patient is the sole driver of decision-making. Most nurses know better. Indeed, they regularly interact with families—who may be from cultures outside the United States—with very different beliefs. People who come from Asian and Hispanic cultures, for instance, often explicitly value family-centered decision-making over patient autonomy.[1] It is important to think through these differences, especially if one identifies as a Christian nurse. There will be times when differences of opinions arise—whether regarding which treatment option is best or who should have a say in making the decision—one must tread a careful path navigating family involvement.[2]

Alisha's experiences led her to believe most nurses have experienced this pull. The calling nurses have is to support their patients, but also the family. Sometimes there is a very cohesive flow, and at other times it is an undulating endeavor in which one has to be aware and respectful of everyone's concerns and role in the care process. Alisha took care of a particularly memorable young patient in the hospital; she was a remarkable young lady, still a teenager, who was dying of cancer. The providers were forthcoming about the patient's fate, but her mother, understandably, could not process or accept it. The patient, however, was facing the reality with fierce courage. In the room, the conversation seemed to avoid any mention of the inevitable. When the mother left for a short time, Alisha decided to sit down and find out how the patient was really doing. They shared a beautiful, honest, vulnerable conversation that will stay with Alisha forever. The young woman said she was ready to face what was to come and that she accepted this fate, but she was holding on to life because she worried about how her mother would be affected once she was gone. It was a burden she did not need to carry in addition to what her young heart had to already deal with. Alisha encouraged her to be open and honest with her mother so they could walk through the end journey together, with full support. The patient's mother was eventually able to have a separate conversation with Alisha—no parent can ever be prepared for that situation, yet one could see a change over the next few weeks before the brave young lady passed away.

An illness or unexpected hospitalization brings with it profound stress and destabilizing uncertainty. During such times, unresolved family tension—or simply differences of opinions on how to proceed—can come to the fore in ways that can be extremely challenging for nurses. What should you do when family members disagree on the direction of care? Or how about when you are treating a minor who is not given a voice in the decision-making process? Or maybe your patient is refusing to share his diagnosis or prognosis with family in an attempt to save them from a burden? The goal is to find a tricky balance between respecting the patient's wishes while also caring for her as a human being who is essentially in relationships with others.

A healthy nurse-patient relationship is crucial for good patient outcomes and for the proper care of the patient. The patient simply must be able to trust that his nurse (and everyone on the medical team) is acting in his best interest and not in the interest of someone or something else. Because we know that the patient's good is essentially bound up in his relationship with others, the nurse's communication and collaboration with those with whom he has relationships (especially his family) is also absolutely essential. There are times, for instance, when patients choose not to be told the details of a diagnosis that might be too painful or overwhelming. Dr. Joseph Clayton, from the University of Sydney, states that patients have different informational needs than their caregivers at certain times. "In that terminal phase," Dr. Clayton says, "caregivers often need more detail about the dying process than the patient. Perhaps the dying person doesn't want to know all about the nitty gritty details about what could go wrong, what to expect in those last days. The caregiver needs that information."[3]

In these kinds of complex situations, nurses must make sure necessary details are provided while respecting the patient's wishes and, again, taking care to prove trustworthy. Patient trust and confidentiality are absolutely crucial for a healthy patient-nurse relationship. This confidentiality provides reassurance to a patient that her private health information is protected, setting the stage for a more intimate and honest conversation. According to patient protection laws, the right to information applies to the individual patient and, if the patient provides consent, to certain family members. However, it is important to remember that health care, especially primary care, is often and ideally provided within the context of the family.[4]

If these goals seem to be in some tension with each other, that's because they often are. There are times in nursing when conflicts arise between protecting a patient's health information, supporting the patient's wishes, and caring for the patient in her context as a member of a family. We will see examples of this as we move to our case study examples below, but here let us pause to keep in mind that this kind of tension is present in the *very nature* of God himself. How can God be one being, one essence, and still be a relationship between three persons? It is a great mystery, full of tension and paradox, but a similar one plays out in the nature and relationships of human beings as well.

CASE STUDY: TWO PATIENTS, TWO FAMILIES, TWO DILEMMAS

We will look at two different case studies that highlight the importance and complexity of the family unit as it intersects with nursing care. Our first case involves a forty-five-year-old patient named Steven, a married man with two teenage children. He is well-known in the community as a dedicated high school football coach. A week before Christmas one year, he came into the emergency room with severe abdominal pain and blood in his stool and was admitted to the hospital for further testing. Initial tests were inconclusive. After consulting with a gastroenterologist, he was informed that they found a tumor growing in his colon—he had colon cancer. He would need further testing to determine the stage of cancer he was battling and to help guide treatment recommendations. The gastroenterologist rounded on the patient first thing in the morning, before his wife came to stay with him for the day. Steven was the only one present for this news. After the physician left, the patient called his wife to tell her not to come to the hospital until later in the day—explaining that he wanted to rest and that he had some more tests to do so would be out of the room.

When the nurse walked in to change his IV fluids, she asked how he was coping with the news. He stated he was still processing it but asked her to put a note in his chart instructing the medical team not to inform his family of the news. Steven said he wanted to figure things out on his own and did not want to burden his family or friends. He had had some vague symptoms for several months that had made him worry that he might have cancer and had decided to protect his wife and children who would not be able to bear the news. The nurse spent several minutes talking with him, but he was adamant on keeping the news private. When his wife and children came to visit, they understandably had a number of questions. Steven's wife even stopped the nurse in the hall to express her frustration that her husband was not getting answers and they were worried about him. The nurse felt torn, and rightly so, between honoring her patient's request while knowing that he was carrying the burden alone and his family could not come together during this time without complete, shared knowledge of the situation.

The second case study looks at the relationship between a nurse and the family unit from a different perspective. We will discuss the patient Maria, a seventy-eight-year-old Spanish-speaking female who was admitted to the hospital for unexplained weight loss and new-onset seizures. She was in remission after a seven-year battle with breast cancer, but now had an unexplained fifteen-pound weight loss and daily headaches. One day after dinner with her daughter, she had a mild seizure. When paramedics brought her to the hospital, a large mass was found in her brain via the CT scan. Maria was still sedated when her family was given the news. Maria's husband had passed away three years prior, but she was extremely close to all three of the children and they were all present for the news. Before anything was shared with their mother, the children requested a family conference with the oncologist and learned that the news was not good. Her cancer was back and had spread to multiple sites. Surgery was not an option and even with chemotherapy, her life expectancy was weeks to months.

Devastated, the children decided together that their mother would not want to know this information and they would bring her home and care for her with palliative care only. Their Hispanic family valued communal decision-making in contexts like these. The attending physician, however, was not comfortable keeping this news from Maria and requested an interpreter be present when he returned in the afternoon so he could talk with the patient. The family became upset at this plan. The nurse, who had been taking care of the patient and comforting the family, felt torn. She knew their wishes were out of care and concern for Maria, but she also understood that the patient had a right to know her medical diagnosis.

CASE ANALYSIS

These two cases approach the principle we are addressing in this chapter in different ways. In the case of Steven, could anyone really say in this case that leaving his family clueless about this situation would be in his best interest? We know that patient outcomes improve dramatically when families are connected to their situation and especially when they are physically present in a patient's attempts to recover.[5] If a medical team chooses to deny Steven's family the chance to be made fully aware of his situation, this may not only harm his family—this may very well harm Steven himself and his chances of surviving colon cancer.

All of this makes perfect sense in the context of a Christian vision of the relational human person. From the very beginning of the Bible God said that "it is not good that man should be alone" and worked to make sure we flourish in relationships with each other. Christians should be the least surprised people on earth to learn that patients do so much better with family fully locked into their situation and supporting them through their difficult time. Christians should also be the least surprised people on earth to learn that Steven's nurse struggled deeply with the idea of refusing to inform his family about his medical situation. Having interacted with Steven and his family, she knew better than perhaps anyone how important it was for his well-being to share the experience and challenges together as a family.

And there is something similar about the case with Maria too, isn't there? As mentioned above, Hispanic families like hers very often reject Western-style individualism in favor of a more relational approach to decision-making. If the medical team decides to tell Maria over the objections of her family, then they not only alienate and agitate the family (likely upsetting Maria in the process); they also deny the wisdom of her family in determining what is best for Maria at this particular moment. If they go ahead and tell Maria that she likely has terminal cancer, then it is too late to achieve whatever goals her family believes are achieved by not directly telling her. In this case it seems to be a peaceful transition to palliative care at home, but one can imagine a slightly different version of this case in which it would be even more dramatic. Suppose that Maria's cancer is advanced but probably curable. And suppose Maria's family insists that her psyche is very fragile and if she is told about her diagnosis she will likely spiral into a deep depression and stop fighting to take steps to get better. For her sake, the family might insist that Maria is not told so as to resist breaking her spirit. Again, telling her the fullness of her diagnosis robs Maria's family of achieving the very good they are setting out to achieve. Once again, the good of the individual cannot be separated from the relationships she has with her family.

That said, there is an important objection to consider here—one which invokes the history of how the US and other Western countries have moved so strongly in support of the radical autonomy of the individual patient. We may lay some of that at the feet of our peculiar historical focus on a "pull yourself up by your own bootstraps" individualist mythology, but most of it comes from terrible excesses of prioritizing the group over the individual. From Nazi eugenics and forced euthanasia, to the Tuskegee syphilis trials, to the (increased) pressure on the old and the sick to make use of assisted suicide, so many of the great ethical abuses we've seen in health care over the last hundred years or so have come when a deeply misguided community violates the inherent, God-given dignity of the individual. Nazi physicians decided that the Third Reich would be better off if the disabled were euthanized. US doctors thought that it was in the interest of Blacks as a community if the syphilis trials were done without full consent of those participating. And today there are a number of health-care providers who believe that the old and sick are better off dead, and thus encourage them to seek assisted suicide. As a result of these kinds of abuses, Western bioethics has understandably focused on protecting individual patient autonomy above almost everything else. Autonomy protects patients from "the many" deciding matters for "the one" in ways that are unjust and deeply harmful—especially when those with power want to enforce a kind of utilitarian calculation which leaves the most vulnerable exposed.

And we don't need to think only about large-scale, utterly horrific historical examples; this concern rings true in more everyday experiences as well. As much as many of those reading this book may love their families, many of these same people likely shield some of their personal decisions so that family doesn't impact them or even know about them. And the reasons for this may range from "Oh my gosh, my mom is just so uptight about stuff like this" to huge areas of profound moral and theological disagreement. Going back to Steven's case, is his medical team really in a place to impose their particular vision of the good onto his situation? Yes, Steven's medical outcome may improve if the family is connected to him and supportive right by his bedside, but how does the medical team know this will be the result if they are told of his situation? Steven obviously knows his family better than his medical team does. What if there is information—and a history—to which they are not privy that would change the calculus? And returning to a situation like Maria's, someone on her medical team might feel comfortable putting the decision in the hands of her family if one were sure they were acting in her patient's best interests. But, again, how can they be sure? What if her family didn't have her best interests in mind and her children were really angling for her life insurance money? Or trying to get out of having to pay for her long-term care? Or what if the loudest members of the family drowned out others who disagreed? These concerns may encourage us to err on the side respecting individual patient autonomy—a very confused place to be, given the major relational thrust of this chapter.

JUDGMENTS INFORMED BY RELATIONSHIPS

There is a deep tension here, or at least there could be. How is contemporary health care supposed to both (1) honor the truth that there really is no such thing as the good of the individual patient apart from his or her relationships with others and (2) acknowledge that attempts to do (1) can often end up going wrong in bad and even horrific ways? Here we believe it is especially important for Christian nurses to acknowledge this tension and paradox—much like, again, the tension and paradox that exists in the doctrine of the Trinity itself. Christians are asked to uphold and live in the tension-filled truth that there is one God in three divine persons. Similarly, we must uphold and live in the tension-filled truth that human beings essentially exist in relationship with each other, while at times acknowledging that it is better to treat them as isolated individuals. This kind of paradox doesn't make for easy decision-making and one-size-fits-all principle-building. It requires getting comfortable with gray areas and uncertainty and with making prudential judgments based on the best information you have at the time. Happily, nurses find themselves in enviable positions with respect to the rest of the medical team when it comes to getting the best information possible about the important relationships in their patients' lives. Nurses are the ones who are most likely to know if the family members are united or divided, if they really have the best interest of the patient in mind, or if the patient's will to keep fighting will likely be broken by difficult news. Christian nurses, especially, should be among the most qualified members of the medical team to inhabit this profoundly difficult space and make informed, prudential judgments about how to handle particular situations.

In our discussion of this topic, and indeed throughout the book, we've seen repeatedly how the theological beliefs and claims Christians make are at the absolute heart of what it means to be a nurse. This, coupled with God's command to love him with everything that we are—our whole selves without remainder—is the subject of the final case-study chapter of our book.

DISCUSSION QUESTIONS

1. This chapter focuses on the importance of relationships in nursing care. Nurses, though having more time to spend with patients than physicians, are increasingly busy during their shifts. This overextended pace can be a threat to relationship building. Given this reality, how can one still build relationships with patients?
2. Nursing often focuses on boundary setting in order to protect oneself from getting too close to patients and to maintain a sense of professionalism. How does one balance building a relationship of true care

for the whole person in the fullness of who they are with the risk of becoming too involved?

3. This chapter makes the provocative claim that, from a Christian point of view, there is really no way to talk about the good for one's patient except in the context of the patient's relationship(s) to others. Do you agree? What complications might this pose for patient care?
4. Often there isn't just one, homogenous family unit to interact with. There are parents, siblings, children, and more. Sometimes these parties disagree with each other. Sometimes they request that you withhold information from another family member or from the patient. How would you handle such disagreements and requests?

11

WITH EVERYTHING THAT WE ARE

> But my life is worth nothing to me unless I use it for finishing the work assigned me by the Lord Jesus—the work of telling others the Good News about the wonderful grace of God.
>
> —*Acts 20:24 (NLT)*

When Jesus gives us the answer to the question "Teacher, which is the greatest commandment in the Law?," it goes without saying that Christians should pay very close attention (see Matt. 22:34–40 NRSV). The command to love the Lord your God with all your heart, all your soul, all your mind, and all your strength is something many of us have heard so often that we may fail to think about what it means for our lives. The command means more than "just really love God a lot." It means being on the lookout for polytheism in our lives. As mentioned in chapter 4, this doesn't involve bowing down before golden idols or offering a pinch of incense to Jupiter or Caesar. Today the concern is about worship of gods like money, sex, and nationalism. The operative word in the commandment Jesus highlights is *all*, which could also be understood as *whole*. For the purpose of this chapter, we will be examining what it means to love God with one's *whole* self. Many Christians love God to a certain extent, or even to a great extent, but still reserve space in their lives for other gods. Jesus's teaching about the greatest commandment makes it crystal clear that there is no such room in the life of a Christian. There are things besides God which are good—in fact, God created them to be good—but our love of those goods needs to be directed to our ultimate and foundational concern: the love of God. We are to love God with everything that we are. Period.

It is helpful to think about our failures to live up to this commandment as a kind of compartmentalization. We manage to live our lives as if, for example, church on Sundays or prayer before meals is in a separate space from our intimate life or our economic practices. Have you ever heard the phrases "It's not personal; it's just business," or "All is fair in love and war," or "What happens in Vegas stays in Vegas"? These are the kinds of attempts to compartmentalize we have in mind here. Normally you would treat someone a certain way, but because we are in this other, separated sphere of life with different rules ("business" or "war" or "romantic relationships") you will be treating someone differently. It is in these other compartmentalized places too many Christians feel pressure to check their Christianity at the door and operate by a different set of values and rules and commands.

Significantly, this has led many Christians to commit some of the worst atrocities of all time. When Nazi soldiers (most of whom identified as Christians) tried to defend and explain their actions they basically offered some version of "I was just doing my job" or "I was just following orders." Nevertheless, the rest of the world rightly held them responsible for crimes against humanity. The underlying lesson here is that—especially when it comes to one's ultimate values—the compartmentalization excuse is no excuse at all. The fundamental respect for human dignity that Nazi soldiers were called to honor (especially as Christians) did not suddenly disappear because of orders they were given or a uniform they were wearing or their chosen profession. We are called to love and honor God, not just with part of ourselves, but with everything that we are. And everything means everything.

Germans like Sister Anna Bertha Königsegg and Catholic nurses working with the disabled, as we saw in chapter 3, had the courage of their convictions in loving God with their whole heart, soul, mind, and strength in an incredibly difficult time and space to do so. They did not let those who had authority over determining what counts as "best practices" or "the standard of care" or "professional behavior" in health care push them to violate their most fundamental values. Happily, though the issues involved are still very significant, the stakes today are much lower for nurses and others working in health care. Nurses working in Nazi Germany could reasonably fear for their lives as a response to loving God with everything that they are. There are important, sometimes even life-changing ramifications for standing up as nurses today—several of which we will discuss in the next chapter—but given that the stakes are significantly lower, then we should expect that even more Christian nurses follow the commandment Jesus told us was the greatest. There is nothing about putting on scrubs, finishing a degree program, or walking through the door of a clinic or hospital which changes the ultimate moral obligations of a Christian nurse. Though there are of course prudential judgments to be made about *how* one loves God with everything that they are, there is no checking that obligation at the door without compartmentalizing one's life in ways that, by definition, honor another god.

NURSES LOVING GOD WITH EVERYTHING THAT WE ARE

For many nurses, their profession is not a space that is cut off from their life as a Christian; rather, it is a central part of that life. Indeed, it is often a profession chosen by Christians precisely because they are Christians. Nurses do the work of Christ like no other profession: they comfort those who are hurting, they help heal wounds (physical and emotional ones), they speak up for those who have no voice, and they show caring, other-centered love toward their vulnerable neighbor. Nurses' physical acts of care—feeding a patient, administering lifesaving medications, holding a hand—are undeniably important to patients' physical healing. No one would question that. But as we've seen throughout this book, there is more to nursing than the physical acts. Nurses don't just help heal the body—they care for patients in the fullness of who they are. Kind words of concern, common acts of prayer, and indeed merely the act of being present can be just as healing for a patient as well. This type of healing converges on the mental, emotional, and spiritual parts of who we are. Today, health-care providers focus almost exclusively on the physical healing—fixing a broken bone, lowering cholesterol levels, or treating an infection. But for deep healing—for *whole patient care*—the focus is on not just physical goods, but emotional, mental, and spiritual goods as well.

Though health care hasn't prioritized such areas historically, the last several years have seen growing interest in the importance of mental and emotional health for the overall good of the patient. Spiritual health, however, does not get talked about nearly enough in the health-care realm. Some of the reasons for this have already been explored in this book—like the idea that authority in medicine comes primarily from technical expertise related to the scientific method. Maybe a health-care provider would agree that mental and emotional health are important, but the assumption is still that medicine is about treating an organic machine. This mindset has led to an underlying belief among some physicians and nurses that discussing spirituality with patients could be considered outside their proper sphere, and therefore unprofessional.

This is deeply unfortunate considering the extremely high percentage of patients who view themselves as religious and even more who identify as spiritual. As we saw in the opening to this book, 84 percent of the world's population identifies with an organized religion. We also saw that the US is disproportionately religious compared to other rich Western countries, with over seven in ten people identifying as Christian. A relatively small number of Americans explicitly say they don't believe in God: ranging from about one in twenty in older people to about one in ten in younger folks. Though younger generations have tended to be more skeptical of religious belief historically, there is a lot of focus on the supposed anti-religiosity of "the nones"—that is, those who claim to have no religious affiliation. Many are seekers with spiritual beliefs that even rise to acknowledgement of transcendent realities.[1] Still more are actually moving in an explicitly religious direction: a recent study, for instance, found that 13 percent more young Catholics say they have become "more religious" over the last five years than young Catholics who say they have become "less religious."[2] It is also important to keep in mind another fact we learned: immigrants and people of color tend to be significantly more religious than native white populations.

Especially in light of these facts, it is clear that health-care teams have a responsibility to acknowledge the important role spiritual health plays in patients' lives. As Danish Zaidi—a former chaplain at Boston Children's Hospital who later went on to medical school—rightly pointed out, "Acknowledging the moral underpinnings (spiritual or religious) that drive certain care-seeking behaviors—from end-of-life care to contraception—is critical in achieving a more holistic medical practice."[3] And spirituality can play an even greater role when patients are hospitalized or facing a serious illness, as many turn toward religion for guidance and support.[4] During times of severe illness, spiritual support from the medical team significantly impacts patient-reported quality of life.[5] And in cases where patients are facing a terminal illness or the end of life, religion and spirituality also improves prognostic acceptance and protects against hopelessness and despair.[6] In one study looking at spiritual care for oncology patients, nearly 80 percent of the patients felt that regular use of spiritual care practices by physicians or nurses would have a positive impact on patients.[7]

Most patients do not receive spiritual care. In another study involving patients with advanced cancer, 87 percent of the oncology nurses and 94 percent of physicians completely ignored their patients' spiritual care.[8] By ignoring this essential part of human life, health care is refusing to address the whole person, and they are even acting in ways which negatively affect physical outcomes. When patients feel their spiritual needs are not met in clinical environments, many are driven away from effective medical treatment. When reviewing the medical records of 172 children who passed away after their parents turned to faith healing instead of traditional medicine, researchers found that most of the children likely would have survived if they also received medical care.[9] Medical care should not be so grossly separated from spiritual care.

The combination of medical care and spiritual care can impact both patient care and patient outcomes. For this reason, the nurse's duty to act on behalf of the patient should include respect for patient spirituality.[10] But what is the spiritual care duty as nurses? Nurses don't often have the same beliefs about these matters as their patients, even if they are fellow Christians. And there are times they don't have the same beliefs as physicians or others on the medical team. To give just one common yet revealing example: case law allows competent patients to withhold or choose treatments based on their religious beliefs, such as when a Jehovah's Witness patient refuses blood products. How should nurses approach a patient with very different beliefs? Well, it doesn't have to be that different than how they treat any other patient—that is, by providing competent and compassionate care with respect to their dignity, which includes their physical and spiritual needs. Asking about their spiritual health and getting permission to incorporate spiritual care is very much part of this. Even when patients are not quite open to it, they can still witness God through nurses' compassion and care. As Edgar A. Guest stated, "I'd rather see a sermon than hear one any day."[11] Or the command often attributed to Saint Francis of Assisi, "Preach the gospel at all times—when necessary, use words."

One powerful example of this is a story that came from the tragic shooting in a Jewish synagogue back in 2018. On October 27, Robert Bowers stormed into the Tree of Life Synagogue, killing eleven people. He was injured in the attack and taken to the local hospital. The nurse who cared for him, Ari Mahler, was Jewish. He later wrote about how and why he showed compassion and empathy to the gunman:

> To be honest, I didn't see evil when I looked into Robert Bowers' eyes. All I saw was a clear lack of depth, intelligence, and palpable amounts of confusion . . . [the gunman] thanked me for saving him, for showing him kindness, and for treating him the same way I treat every other patient. I'm sure he had no idea I was Jewish . . . Love. That's why I did it. Love as an action is more powerful than words, and love in the face of evil gives others hope. It demonstrates humanity. It reaffirms why we're all here.[12]

These words are beautiful and they demonstrate how powerful love can be. In that moment, Ari did not separate his religion from his profession. He approached the patient as both a caring nurse and a man of faith. It is through these actions that patients and communities can heal. There will be times that you as a nurse will be put in difficult situations where your Christian faith and nursing obligations intersect in a tension-filled way. Let us now focus on a case study in which a nurse's actions were put into question in the midst of precisely this kind of tension.

CAROLINE PRAYING WITH HER PATIENTS

For many nurses and patients alike, prayer is an extremely common practice—the lifeblood of one's relationship with the divine. Unsurprisingly, very large majorities of Americans pray during a typical week.[13] Naturally, Christian nurses very often want to incorporate prayer into the overall care for their patients. But as Caroline Petrie found out the hard way, prayer is not always welcomed by the patient or even permitted by the organization for which a nurse works. Caroline is a Christian registered nurse who made a 2008 home visit to a female patient in Somerset, England. This was the first time meeting the patient. At the end of the visit, Caroline asked the patient a question that was part of her routine care: "Would you like me to pray for you?" The patient declined and Caroline respected the patient's wishes and left.

After the visit was over, however, the patient called Caroline's employer, North Somerset Trust, and reported the incident. She stated that although the prayer offer did not upset her, she was concerned that it could upset other patients.[14] North Somerset decided to suspend Caroline. She was accused of breaching the code of conduct by using her professional status to "promote causes that are not related to health" and by failing to "demonstrate a personal and professional commitment to equality and diversity."[15] She was later allowed to return to work, but this case brought international attention. *The Nursing Times* even conducted a survey and received over 2,500 respondents in three days. The large majority of people (91 percent) sided with Caroline.[16] There were a few who felt she overstepped her boundaries by offering prayer without the patient first requesting it.

PRUDENTIAL JUDGMENTS WITHOUT SIDELINING FAITH

Many Christian nurses—at least those who do not compartmentalize their values—can empathize with Caroline's approach. Their work as nurses is part of their ministry. So how can they be asked to take their Christian hat off at the door before entering the patient's room? As Dr. Elizabeth Johnston Taylor stated in *The Journal of Christian Nursing*:

> How does the Christian nurse juxtapose an inner mandate to "preach the gospel" everywhere with a professional ethic for clinical practice that may caution or prevent such preaching? This raises an important question: Should spiritual care include Christians sharing their faith (i.e., evangelism)? Might there be a possibility that the "good news" could be perceived as bad news when it is introduced by a nurse to a patient?[17]

Alisha herself has personal experience with this topic. She was a Christian before becoming a nurse, and like so many Christian nurses, her faith is what led her to nursing. She worked in several settings over the years—in some secular practices and even in a Catholic hospital—but often brought spirituality into her care of patients. But, like Caroline, Alisha always used discernment and prudential judgment when doing so, including always asking the patient's permission to provide spiritual care. This allows one to find out more about where patients are and invite them to become drivers of the conversation. If a patient declines the offer or makes it clear they are not spiritual, then one should obviously respect their choice. But the majority of Alisha's patients appreciate the conversation and want to include faith as part of their health care. Indeed, opportunities to comfort countless patients during difficult times with spiritual discussions or prayer has been one of the greatest privileges of Alisha's nursing profession. These opportunities not only allow Christian nurses to live out what they fundamentally believe to be true, they actually allow us to be better nurses by forming deeper connections with patients and thus opening up more opportunities for empathy and building trust. Nurses who engage the spiritual reality of patients very often find out more about the fullness of their reality in ways that make their care that much better.

Prudential judgment is required to balance various goods here. A clinical setting—like many other places in life—is not a place for proselytizing. It is one thing to invite the patient to take the lead in how far to pursue spiritual matters, but it is obviously not a good idea to force prayer or another spiritual exchange on patients who don't want it. In such cases, a Christian nurse can preach the gospel with something other than words. One of the most attractive things about the early church was the great love that Christians showed others. "See how they love one another!" was the line the church father Tertullian related to those attracted to the Jesus movement.[18] Nurses have a paradigmatic opportunity to demonstrate the attractiveness of Christian care and love. Forcing prayer or formal attempts to convert a patient are not only professionally inappropriate in a clinical setting—they actually distract from the true power of the gospel.

FOUNDATIONAL BELIEFS AND THE RELIGIOUS FREEDOM OF NURSES

But what about other contexts in which ultimate concerns are in play—like the Jehovah's Witness example suggested above? Suppose a patient wants to get an organ transplant or other similar procedure without blood products? Here, also, there can be a prudential judgment made about how to balance certain goods and approaches. One would not have to agree with this aspect of the procedure, of course, to participate in it and try to do one's best for the good of the patient.[19] But if we are going to honor the foundational reasons so many religious people become nurses, we need to protect their ability to act (or not act) on the basis of their foundational beliefs. If religious nurses cannot participate in good conscience in a procedure that they believe requires a blood transfusion, they should be able to opt out. No one should force them to go against their foundational beliefs. And this is true of other kinds of cases where foundational issues of human dignity are at stake as well, some of which we've already encountered: abortion, assisted suicide, eugenic practices in reproduction, and more.

Not everyone agrees that the religious freedom of nurses should be protected this way, however. Indeed, a shift to a kind of vending machine style of medicine—in which patients simply expect to get whatever they choose from on demand—suggests that the religious freedom of nurses is under serious threat. In the final three chapters of the book, we will look at the future of nursing, and we begin by focusing on what is coming down the pike when it comes to protecting nurse consciences.

DISCUSSION QUESTIONS

1. This chapter provided data showing that many nurses and physicians completely ignore their patients' spiritual care, despite patients wanting these needs addressed. What are the reasons for this? What are potential solutions to try to overcome this gap in patient care?
2. Think about the British nurse Caroline praying with her patients. What are the potential pitfalls in praying with patients? How should one respond to a patient who asks for prayer?
3. Do you feel comfortable praying with patients? Why or why not? Have you had any personal experiences praying with patients?

PART THREE

The Future of a Profession on the Move

12

PROTECTING NURSE CONSCIENCES

> Freedom of conscience, religious freedom, the freedom of each person, each family, each people, is what gives rise to rights.
>
> – *Pope Francis*

If Christians are to be the kinds of nurses who can fully honor the duty to love God with everything that they are (including and especially through their vocation caring for vulnerable patients) it goes without saying that they must be professionally and legally free to do so. Asking them to check the greatest of all commandments at the door of the clinic means asking them to check the deepest part of themselves at the door as well. Any plausible attempt to respect the dignity of the human person must also respect his seeking to make his way in the world such that he can align his life with the fundamental values he holds most dear. Such values, the Catholic Church notes, are ones he has discovered in his conscience, which is "the most secret core and sanctuary of a man." It is in one's conscience where God's voice "echoes in his depths."[1]

Respecting such a profoundly sacred space is an essential part of what it means to show broad respect for basic, fundamental human rights. This includes the right to pursue and respond to one's individual relationship with God. But very often it also helps to produce good and just outcomes as well. Obviously, the nurses and physicians who resisted the violent eugenic programs of Nazi medicine discussed in chapter 3 are paradigmatic examples of this. Also revealing is the inspiring story of Dawn Wooten from chapter 8, an African American nurse with the courage of her deepest convictions and experiences to blow the whistle on the racist and xenophobic injustices being done to undocumented detainees. God's voice echoed in her secret core, the most profound depths of who she is, and she acted on those profound convictions in ways that exposed practices that were horrifically discriminatory.

But we should not forget the negative reactions Wooten faced from her institution because she acted on her values. Too often nurses are still thought of as mere cogs in the wheel of institutional medicine—assistants who are expected to go along and get along and not rock the boat. On this view, it is those who hold power within health-care institutions (which, as we will see below, some consider to be patients) who decide what the right thing is to do in any given situation, regardless of the views of individual providers of care. In this chapter we are deeply concerned that this view is ascendant in our dominant secular medical culture—a culture which finds it increasingly difficult to even make sense of religious freedom, much less make it a priority. Once considered "the first freedom," it is now under serious threat and in need of an intense and robust defense, especially for nurses who don't have the same power as physicians and others who can effect change on the health-care team.

THE CONTEMPORARY SITUATION

In setting up the reasons for our concern, it just so happens that perhaps the paradigmatic contemporary case of what we believe is coming down the pike involves the coercion of a religious nurse. According to coverage by the *Atlantic* of a complaint filed in May of 2018, a Catholic nurse with a longstanding public objection to participating in abortion procedures was actually tricked into participating in one.[2] Despite being on a list of objectors, she was scheduled for what she was told was a procedure following a miscarriage when it was actually an elective abortion. According to the complaint, the attending physician said, "Don't hate me" when the nurse became aware of how she was tricked. Fearing retaliation based on a policy that could punish staffers who refuse to participate when they are short-staffed, the nurse did participate in the abortion.

The Office of Civil Rights (OCR) with Health and Human Services investigated the complaint but did not receive cooperation from the Vermont Medical Center where this nurse was working. As part of their investigation, OCR found that this was not an isolated incident for the medical center. Indeed, OCR spoke with "several" other health-care personnel who had been "intentionally, unnecessarily, and knowingly scheduled by the University of Vermont Medical Center (UVMMC) to assist with elective abortions against their religious or moral objections." Like the nurse who filed the complaint, many of these other personnel were not told in advance that they were going to participate in an abortion. Quite rightly, OCR argued that when health-care staff are put into situations like these, they "suffer moral injury, are subjected to a crisis of conscience, and frequently experience significant emotional distress, even if they succeed in declining to assist in the procedure after the assignment is made."[3]

Nor are these kinds of practices limited to this particular medical center. In 2017, the Alliance Defense Fund filed a lawsuit against Mt. Sinai Hospital in New York on behalf of another Catholic nurse who "was forced to participate in a late-term abortion under the threat of disciplinary action, including possible termination and loss of her license."[4] And the concern is most certainly not limited to nurses. Dr. Regina Frost, an OB-GYN and member of the Christian Medical and Dental Associations, leads a network of health-care professionals called Women Physicians in Christ. Called to care for their patients "like Christ would," they are explicitly approaching their health-care ministry from the deepest parts of who they are.[5] But at the time we are writing, the state of New York is actually suing the OCR at Health and Human Services so that Dr. Frost and others like her are forced to perform procedures that grossly violate their consciences.[6]

This kind of force is also being used in medical schools and residency programs. In California, for instance, residency programs in obstetrics and gynecology must comply with the program requirements set by the Accreditation Council for Graduate Medical Education, which includes training in "the performance of abortion services."[7] There are even articles published in the *New England Journal of Medicine* which argue that, if Catholic and other religiously affiliated hospitals become too prominent in a given area, they should be legally compelled to provide "certain health services," even if it fundamentally violates their religious mission.[8] And though what they mean by "services" here certainly includes abortion, it increasingly means physician-assisted killing as well. California, which legalized such killing back in 2015 on the basis of not interfering with the autonomy of patients, is already interfering with the autonomy of providers by forcing them to participate in it in ways that violate their consciences. Indeed, if religious providers decide that they don't want to participate in such killings, California is trying to compel them to make sure their patients do find a doctor who will help kill them.[9]

What about providers with a religious objection to participating in such a task? A court in Ontario, Canada, responded rather bluntly to this idea: "It would appear that, for these [objecting] physicians, the principal, if not the only, means of addressing their concerns would be a change in the nature of their practice if they intend to continue practicing medicine in Ontario."[10] In other words, for religious health-care providers, if you are going to choose this profession, certain parts of it simply won't be open to you. You may *wish* to be an oncologist and care for cancer patients, but if you aren't willing to participate in them killing themselves then you'll need to find another place to work. This is also the position of Ezekiel Emanuel, one of the chief architects of the Affordable Care Act and important advisor to the Biden administration. He claims (also in the *New England Journal of Medicine*[11]) that those with religious objections can either choose an area of health care that isn't impacted all that much by one's faith or simply avoid becoming a health-care provider in the first place. The influential Canadian bioethicist Udo Schuklenk offered a similar view in an article he published with the *Journal of Medical Ethics* titled: "Professionalism Eliminates Religion as a Proper Tool for Doctors Rendering Advice to Patients."[12] Indeed, Schuklenk would want to facilitate this cultural change by barring people with religious views he doesn't like from medical, nursing, and pharmacy schools.[13]

Things do not look good for protecting the consciences of Christian nurses and other health-care providers. Indeed, President Biden's choice for Secretary of Health and Human Services, Xavier Becerra, was asked at a confirmation hearing about how he used his position as Attorney General of California to force all groups, even churches, to cover abortion in the health insurance they offered their employees.[14] Attempts to protect the consciences of health-care workers during the Trump administration are also being challenged by the politically powerful Planned Parenthood Federation of America—and as this challenge winds its way through the courts, it would do well for Christian nurses to note that it singles out religious beliefs for special critical scrutiny.[15]

STANDING UP FOR CONSCIENCE PROTECTIONS

It is not *the first* reason, but one of the most important reasons Christian nurses should feel confident in asserting their rights of conscience—despite all this opposition—is that outside of the power structures mentioned above there is broad support for health-care providers to exercise their right of conscience. And these come from far outside any recognizable Christian body. According to the World Medical Organization, for instance, "No physician should be forced to participate in euthanasia or assisted suicide, nor should any physician be obliged to make referral decisions to this end."[16] The American Medical Association very strongly supports conscience rights, voting for new policies in 2014 that made this support even more clear.[17] They affirmed, among other things, that the right of conscience exists when "an action will undermine the physician's personal integrity" or "create emotional or moral distress for the physician." They even went so far as to say that a physician can "decline to refer" when the matter involves "a deeply held, well-considered personal belief." On the issue of abortion, in *Doe v. Bolton* (the companion case to *Roe v. Wade*), the Supreme Court of the United States left a law in place that insisted "a physician or any other employee has the right to refrain, for moral or religious reasons, from participating in the abortion procedure."[18] In addition, the 2004 Hyde/Weldon Conscience Protection Amendment protects physicians and nurses, hospitals, health insurance companies, and other health-care entities from being forced by state or federal governments to perform, pay for, provide coverage of, or refer for abortions. At the time of this writing, it has been approved every year since 2004. The federal office of Health and Human Services also insists that a health-care provider may file a complaint under "Federal Health Care Provider Conscience Protection Statutes" if the provider believes they have experienced discrimination because they

1. Objected to, participated in, or refused to participate in specific medical procedures, including abortion and sterilization, and related training and research activities

2. Were coerced into performing procedures that are against your religious or moral beliefs
3. Refused to provide health care items or services for the purpose of causing, or assisting in causing, the death of an individual, such as by assisted suicide or euthanasia.[19]

Unsurprisingly, especially given what we learned about the Catholic understanding of conscience above, the Catholic Church has a very strong support for conscience in health care. Indeed, the United States Conference of Catholic Bishops has a whole office and set of institutional structures set up to defend religious freedom, and a significant part of this is set up to address the health-care context.[20] Nor does this come from simply the "conservative" side of the Catholic Church, as Pope Francis himself has spoken forcefully in support of religious freedom and conscience protection. Indeed, the Pope said that "freedom of conscience and religious freedom—which is not limited to freedom of worship alone, but allows all to live in accordance with their religious convictions—are inseparably linked to human dignity."[21] And in case one was uncertain about just how important this issue is for him, he has claimed that conscientious objection is a basic human right.[22]

Evangelical Christians are also very committed to protecting religious freedom in health care, with the appropriately-titled "Ethics and Religious Liberty Commission" being one of the most important leaders in this fight.[23] The Christian Medical and Dental Associations are deeply concerned, especially given their grounding in Scripture, about complicity with evil.[24] "This complicity," they argue, "may involve using, rewarding, perpetuating, justifying, or ignoring past or present evil." It may also involve "enabling or facilitating future immoral actions of patients or professionals." They also note that protecting conscience in health care is not only about human rights, but also about preserving a diversity of views within the field of medicine itself.[25] When we tell a Christian nurse she may not participate in some fields of health care based on her foundational beliefs, we not only violate her human rights—we also do damage to one of the most important concepts in medicine (indeed, in most fields of knowledge): a free and open exchange of diverse ideas.

Indeed, Christians who care both about human rights and the good of the medical field should be defending not only our own rights of conscience but also those of non-Christians and secular folks as well. We should be aiming to protect these rights when an Orthodox Jew refuses to treat a brain-dead patient as if they have actually died.[26] We should also be supportive of a Muslim who wants to honor the traditional Islamic belief that patients should only be seen by a provider of the same sex.[27] And because this issue is one of fundamental human rights, it would also apply to a secular nurse who doesn't want to participate in an abortion.[28]

NOT JUST DEFENDING RIGHTS, BUT PRODUCING GOOD CONSEQUENCES

Especially given some of the insights that we have been at pains to express about the deep insight nurses have—both about their patients specifically and health care in general—it would be surprising if empowering nurses this way didn't produce good consequences. We've seen several examples of this already, including the aforementioned Dawn Wooten and the German nurses who resisted Nazi euthanasia programs. And even though the primary reason to afford nurses conscience protection comes from a defense of their human rights, it is still worth noting in even more detail just how much good such a defense can accomplish.

Consider, for instance, the following example. During the COVID-19 pandemic, a study of those working in care homes in the United Kingdom found that a whopping "[t]hirty-four percent of people working in health and/or social care said they were under pressure to put DNACPRs [do not attempt cardiopulmonary resuscitation orders] in place without involving the person."[29] Yes, you read that correctly: more than one in three claimed that they were under pressure to put orders in place not to revive a person without the consent of the person herself. And who do you think blew the whistle? Nurses, of course. Indeed, the Queen's Nursing Institute claimed based on their data that the "decisions were being made by NHS [National Health Service] managers, not clinicians. And this wasn't just happening with elderly people, it was those with learning disabilities or cognitive problems of all ages."[30] And beyond the fact that they weren't discussed with the patients/residents themselves, nurses also complained about resuscitation decisions made by general practitioners, hospital staff, or clinical commissioning groups given that these decisions were also often without the input of "families or care home staff" or that they "disagreed with some of the decisions on legal, professional or ethical grounds."[31]

Now, to be clear, we can also imagine some critics of our defense of religious freedom and conscience protection because, on their view, they actually produce bad consequences. There are some who will say that such a strong defense of conscience will sometimes harm patients who want certain things done that certain health-care providers won't do. And while rare, especially in an urban context when there are plenty of health-care options, defenders of conscience should admit that this may in fact be the case. There may in fact be delays in the scheduling of procedures or longer commutes for patients if certain health-care providers are not forced to participate in ways that violate the core part of who they are. But there are at least two important things to think about in response to this concern. First, whether what takes place is in fact a harm or a benefit relies on the vision of the good that one brings to the table in evaluating it. From our Christian perspective, if no one can be found to do an elective abortion because nurses or others are refusing, that is very much a good consequence, not a bad one.

Second, we must think about the consequences for the profession of health care itself if we fail to protect the consciences of health-care providers in relation to their patients. Even describing health care as a profession implies that there are certain rules or norms that the professionals determine as a field. It is not like a vending machine where you simply push a button and get whatever you want—profession determines the objective facts about the norms and goals of its practices. If patients can simply demand of health-care providers whatever they like, then this fundamentally changes the model of what health care is. Unlimited patient demand changes health care from an ends-based, professional, and objective practice to, essentially, just another kind of market transaction in which customers are always right. This would be a transition in which customers can compel health-care providers to provide products in whatever way the customer sees fit. If this kind of approach becomes normalized, health care as an objective profession ceases to exist. And the negative consequences of this happening are so vast that they are impossible to calculate.

Thank God, literally, that nurses we've discussed in this chapter and elsewhere in this book felt empowered to speak up. But let's be honest: the place and power of nurses should go beyond reporting what has happened in a survey or study. It should not be, as some nurses have found out the hard way, that a nurse can put her job at risk for speaking up based on her foundational beliefs. We believe a significant part of the problem here is that nurses are not really seen as full members of the health-care team. Too often they are thought of as merely assistants rather than as co-equals to physicians, pharmacists, specialists, and other health-care providers who are working for the good of the patient.

Given what we have discussed in this chapter—from empowering nurse consciences to having a coherent idea of what health care is—it is past time to demand that nurses take their rightful places on health-care teams. And this change is the topic of our next chapter.

DISCUSSION QUESTIONS

1. We live in an era in which those with power are increasingly skeptical of religious freedom. How should Christian nurses respond when asked to do something that is in violation of their conscience in the setting of their vocation?
2. Promoting conscience in health care is often framed as an issue that limits choices for patients and is a way for people of faith to "control" or "prevent" people from accessing care or services that are legal in the United States. How would you respond to this criticism? Can the religious freedom of providers be reframed in a more positive way?
3. What direction do you think health care is going with respect to the protection of health-care workers' consciences? Are you concerned or hopeful for future protection?

13

THE RIGHTFUL PLACE OF NURSES ON HEALTH-CARE TEAMS

Nursing is a progressive art such that to stand still is to go backwards.

– *Florence Nightingale*

We have covered many topics so far in this book, from the history of nursing to current nursing ethical dilemmas. We have talked about what it means to be a nurse, and specifically, what it means to be a Christian nurse. A point we've tried to emphasize several times now is that the role of the nurse goes well beyond technical expertise and focuses on care for the whole person—and for Christians (along with other spiritual people), this means not only the body and mind, but the spirit as well. And we have discussed what exactly the theological vision of nursing encompasses throughout the book. Human beings are made in the image and likeness of their creator. All human beings are equal, not based on this or that trait, but rather as fellow living human beings with a shared dignified nature. The Christian nurse understands this and, as we presented in chapter 4, guides his care through this understanding: "Christian nurses are called not only to bind up the wounds of the patient, but in the spirit of mercy to be physically close to them in their illness. . . . This kind of care—

at which nurses are so skilled—has physical benefits for patients to be sure, but it also has spiritual ones. It respects the fullness of the dignity of the human being who, again, was created to be in relationships with others."

And while nursing has seen many different changes over the centuries, the core of what nursing is has stayed the same—a profession that provides compassionate and effective care to those in need. The World Health Organization captures much of what nurses do beautifully:

> Nursing encompasses autonomous and collaborative care of individuals of all ages, families, groups and communities, sick or well and in all settings. It includes the promotion of health, the prevention of illness, and the care of ill, disabled and dying people. Nurses play a critical role in health care and are often the unsung heroes in health care facilities and emergency response. They are often the first to detect health emergencies and work on the front lines of disease prevention and the delivery of primary health care, including promotion, prevention, treatment and rehabilitation.[1]

And just as important as it is to protect the core of what nursing is, it is also important to allow the profession's growing edge to evolve. As the opening quote from Nightingale insists: nursing is a progressive art and standing still is going backwards. In this chapter, we are insisting that one essential way for nurses to influence patient care and health-care delivery systems is for nurses to take their rightful place on health-care teams. As we discussed in chapter 2, nurses make up the largest group of professionals in health care; without nurses, there would be no health-care system. But it is not just a matter of numbers. Because of their particular calling to care for the whole person, and especially the whole person *in relationship*, nurses taking their rightful place on health-care teams would lead to significant improvements in patient care as well as the delivery of health-care services. This is especially true given what we've learned in the last several years about social determinants of health and the need to promote health care over disease care. In fact, as you will see below, it is not too strong to suggest that we are moving toward a new vision of health care—one in which nurses will be quite ready to take intensely important roles.

A CALL FOR NURSES

The United States is facing a complicated dilemma—one which has no end in sight, at least if we merely maintain the status quo. Health-care costs, as well as morbidity and chronic diseases, are on the rise. In fact, overall health-care costs are anticipated to rise by an average of 5.5 percent per year over the next several years, growing from $3.5 trillion in 2017 to $6 trillion by 2027. Furthermore, health-care spending is projected to increase faster than the economy, growing from 17.9 percent of the gross domestic product (GDP) in 2017 to 19.4 percent by 2027.[2] Because of these issues, the pressures on and complexity of the health-care system have increased dramatically over the last several years. Both of these, coupled with growing awareness of patients' medical and care needs, have led to more and more systematic thinkers to demand that nurses play a greater role in guiding the direction of health care.[3] In fact, the Institute of Medicine (IOM) has publicly called upon nurses to lead efforts toward health-care change.[4] This call for nurse leadership actually began several years ago when data could no longer hide the fact that the health-care system was broken.

One of the key turning points in health care was the 1999 publication of the IOM report titled *To Err Is Human: Building a Safer Health System.*[5] The report took a deep dive into the structures and systems by which the United Stated delivered health care—focusing in particular on the errors that were made and the cost related to those errors.[6] The numbers were alarming. The report stated that errors caused up to 98,000 deaths in American hospitals each year and resulted in over one million injuries.[7] We were missing the mark in keeping patients safe and preventing unnecessary disease and suffering. Fast forward to 2015 when the IOM published *The Future of Nursing: Leading Change, Advancing Health*, once again calling on nurses to take a lead role in improving nursing, as well as the health-care system at large. Many of the reasons for this can be attributed to the gap that we see in health care from evidence to practice. Before the monumental publication of *To Err Is Human*, health care was often grounded merely in the opinion and institution of those who held power and simply what every provider had been doing for a very long time. But over the last two decades there has been a push to shift health care from the older model to one held strictly to what are called evidence-based practices (EBP). Unfortunately, on average, it takes about seventeen years to move research findings into clinical practice—a major reason for the delay in implementing these findings.[8] Furthermore, incorporating evidence-based frameworks and practices increases the complexity of health-care delivery, which requires even more education and training in order to fruitfully deliver better care under this model.[9]

So why the push for nurses to lead the change here? Nurses are the ones at the bedside! They see the needs firsthand and they witness patient outcomes in real time. Nurses make direct observations about the needs related to patient outcomes. Rather than relying on the intuitions of powerful people, or doing things only the way they have always been done, nursing observations and experiences provide absolutely essential evidence to guide research and make practices more effective. Indeed, nurses are by far the most valuable component toward moving to EBP care. Also, the more we learn about treating disease—and, even more foundationally, keeping people healthy—it becomes essential to note that nurses practice holistic care. An evidence-based approach means that we can no longer address the complex health needs of our nation by chasing diseases. We must take a step back and approach the health of our nation in a holistic manner—something nurses know a great deal about.

A NEW VISION OF HEALTH CARE

Health care is changing. Patients are living longer and with more chronic diseases than they did in the centuries before. In addition, technology is advancing at a rapid pace. These changes require a different approach to address the needs of individual patients, as well as population health. Health-care changes require a proactive stance. Health-care structures and teams must prepare for the future by anticipating patient needs, thinking about potential obstacles, and then finding nimble and even innovative ways to address them. One proven way to do this is through whole-person, patient- and relationship-centered care. It is not an exaggeration to say that a shift in this direction is fundamentally changing the nature of medicine and its relationship to health care.

A patient-centered model of care insists that patients play a greater role in their care. "Patient-centered care" is a term itself that has been around for years, but is becoming more of a focus as health care transforms from a top-down model from provider to patient and focuses more on the relationship between the two. For years, a paternalistic model of medicine started with the fact that the provider had the knowledge so he or she should make the decision about what is best for the patient. Those on the leading edge of contemporary health-care trends are moving away from this practice and putting the relationship with the patient—the whole patient (including her beliefs and values)—at the center. A patient should have a primary voice in her health-care journey.

A crucial step in the direction of this goal is getting away from a term that is used too often by members of many health-care teams: "noncompliant patient." When a patient is unsuccessful with meeting "our" goals and following through with "our" plans, they are termed noncompliant. In taking this approach, however, health-care teams miss a critical opportunity. Rather than labeling them we need to pull in closer to the fullness of their whole situation. What were the reasons they did not follow through with the plan? Were they even part of the planning process to begin with? Do they have the resources and understanding to follow through? Is there a need that is unmet that could make them more successful to reach their goals? When we take into consideration the patient as a whole—their desires, values, resources, understanding, environment—we can create a plan together that leads the patient toward better health and wellness. This is whole-person care. This is a new vision of health care. As Dr. Susan Mazer eloquently puts it:

> The concept of aiming at wholeness, in spite of a condition that may or may not be curable, is foreign to a system that is married to quantitative measures and reimbursement. However, the high cost, both human and economic, of a society that is unwell in so many ways but only treatable when curing is inevitable, is no longer affordable. Whole Person Care allows the humanity of patient and caregiver to enter into the intimate relationship needed to get well and stay well. It sees the physical, behavioral, and social needs of a single patient as part of a whole system, with each perspective contributing to the long-term outcome.[10]

And there's another evidence-based insight: you don't get whole-person care without intense focus on what have been called social determinants of health (SDOH). When a health-care team focuses on SDOH they are explicitly aware of economic, cultural, religious, environmental, and other social factors which very much impact a patient's health.[11] Particular attention should be given to social status, income, education, and the local community in which a person lives—all of which can affect access to health care, transportation, safety, affordable housing, and many other factors related to the overall health of the patient.[12] Nurses, it should now go without saying, are uniquely positioned to focus on how a particular patient—in relationship with their family and others—is affected by SDOH. By focusing on these sets of concerns moving forward, health-care systems and teams can help create physical and social environments that promote health and wellness for all.[13] This will require collaboration by nurses, physicians, policy makers, and communities, of course. But nurses are in the position to lead this movement and create lasting change that not only improves medicine and health care, but also works toward disease prevention and healthier communities overall.

INTERPROFESSIONAL COLLABORATION AND THE NURSE'S VOICE

The Robert Wood Johnson Foundation released a report titled *Activating Nursing to Address Unmet Need in the 21st Century*, which yes, called on nurses to take the lead in creating collaborative partnerships in moving toward this new model of health care. According to one of the authors, Dr. Pittman, "There is a growing recognition that medical care alone is insufficient to address growing health problems of today's world. Nurses are uniquely positioned to coordinate partnerships and provide . . . holistic, patient- and relationship-centered care."[14] These partnerships, including interprofessional collaboration, can improve the delivery and outcome of patient care. The evidence shows that interprofessional collaboration improves patient outcomes and decreases health-care costs.[15]

Unfortunately, it is not uncommon for competition to exist between, as well as within, roles in health care, with insecure members of the team more concerned about pecking order and prestige—more concerned with peacocking in ways that demonstrate that their role is superior and of greater importance for patient care.[16] It is an unfortunate reality between the different professions, but also within nursing staff. This approach, needless to say, creates barriers to achieving the goal of whole-person care. Alisha has witnessed this several times over the years. She witnessed incivility toward new nurses. She also saw friction between nurses and physicians. She saw patients go without adequate pain medication because nurses were too afraid to call certain physicians due to their unpleasant personalities. One patient she cared for was declining, but when she paged the surgeon, he ignored her concerns and told her not to page him again. Alisha had to page the surgeon a couple more times before he agreed to come and assess the patient. By the time he arrived, the patient was not doing well at all.

And even as an advanced practice nurse, Alisha has received very mixed responses toward her role. She has been very fortunate to work with physicians and staff who have understood and appreciated the role of the nurse practitioner. She has worked closely with many physicians and other advanced practice nurses who model what respectful, cooperative communication looks like. And she has seen how much better patient care is because of these working relationships. And unfortunately, she has also experienced a disregard for her role. Here she recalls a patient she saw at her family practice clinic:

> I was seeing a middle-aged man in an acute appointment for a rash. He had already been seen by one of the providers in our office and the emergency room for the same rash. He was treated for scabies both times. He was clearly agitated and fidgeted in the seat. He believed that he had a rare form of scabies that were resistant to treatment and was having trouble sleeping from it. The more I talked to him, the more concerned I became by his behavior. He did not have the normal presentation of scabies. He had no itching, his wife and

> children did not have any symptoms, and he simply did not have the normal presentation of the condition. He then tried to show me "a moving bug" in his leg while he kept picking at his skin. I was certain that he was dealing with psychosis. He was under the care of a psychiatrist for depression and anxiety and right before this "rash" appeared, he had started on a new medication. I was concerned that he was either experiencing an adverse reaction to his new medication, or that the psychiatrist was missing his true diagnosis. I called the psychiatrist's office to speak to him about the patient. When he got on the phone and found out I was a nurse practitioner, he asked to speak to the doctor instead of me. I explained that the physician did not see this patient and was not aware of the situation. He insisted, and I pulled the physician out of a room so the two of them could talk. Unfortunately, although not surprisingly, the physician could not answer any of the psychiatrist's questions about the patient. After about ten minutes of wasted time, the physician I worked with advised him to talk to me to get a better report. He agreed, but it was very clear during the call that he did not respect my opinion or judgment. He did agree to see the patient in his office for further evaluation. I am not sure of the outcome of that visit, but I hope that the disrespect for my role did not prevent the patient from receiving appropriate care.

As previously stated, we see disrespect among nurses themselves. There are seasoned nurses who have a reputation for what is termed "eating their young." This incivility is a major concern and a cause for some new nurses to actually leave the profession. If nurses are pushing for respect from other professions, they also need to make sure they are leading by example.

Physicians, community members, nurses, nurse practitioners, psyche evaluators, social workers, chaplains—that is, everyone on the health-care team—must acknowledge the essential roles of everyone involved in order for interprofessional collaboration to occur and move toward safe and effective patient care.[17] Input from everyone must be sought, heard, and respected. Visions that are created and practiced in silos are dysfunctional and can lead to organizational failure.[18] Traditionally, it must be said, medical decision-making not only left the patient out, it left out some of the most important voices on the health-care team. Nurses, who observe the evidence firsthand, are often left out of positions to promote change. They see how nurse-patient ratios directly affect patient outcomes, but the leaders making the decisions about staffing needs are individuals removed from bedside care. Nurses see certain treatment protocols being utilized that are inefficient and ineffective, yet they have no say in whether these protocols are changed. Decisions are made from the top down without those at the top receiving any input from those who spend the most time in direct patient care—which seems like the biggest oversight in the traditional health-care model.

It is absolutely imperative for nurses to find their voices on health-care teams. This calls for nurses, health-care organizations, and the health-care system as a whole to recognize and appreciate the value nurses bring to the health-care team, which is the central argument of this chapter. Nurses must be at the decision-making table speaking on behalf of patients, the profession, and even the overall direction in which health care should go. If we are going to achieve goals when it comes to patient- and relationship-centered, whole-person care, the current hierarchy in health care must be restructured to allow for a more inclusive approach to evidence presentation and even ultimate decision-making. To the extent that there is a hierarchy at all, it must be one where there is a genuine team which—though making space for disagreement—has the same generalized vision, the same overall goals, and (most importantly) genuine and mutual respect for one another's input, especially the patient's position, which is often the last consideration.

This shift should occur at both the micro and the macro levels: bedside nursing, the health-care team, ethics committees, public health, and health-care policy development. Nurses should be advocating for these changes to occur now. Not next year. Not next week. *Now*. Advocacy is the first step toward helping to lead to the kind of change promised by the current trajectory under the new model. If nurses don't use their voices to push for necessary changes, then, frankly, other groups will come forth and speak on nurses' behalf. And those voices do not have the profession of nursing's best interest or the patient's care needs in mind.[19] It is the *voices of nurses* that will have the greatest impact in these areas. And it is long past time for them to be heard as co-equal members of the health-care team.

THE VOICE OF THE CHRISTIAN NURSE

The need to step up is no less present for the Christian nurse. In fact, it is even more so given the shift in health care. Christian nurses must be vocal about their commitment to their ministry and protecting their rights, or others will be very happy to make decisions for them on how they practice their ministry and their art of caring. Just as health care has changed over the years, so has the type of ethical situations nurses are faced with, as discussed throughout this book. Physicians and nurses alike once considered it their sacred duty to protect their patients' lives, relieve pain, and promote wellness. Today some actively take—or assist in the taking of—human life. Some of the changes we have seen over the last several decades have altered the face of medicine, blurring what it means to be a nurse or physician.[20] The Christian foundation of health care has slowly been filed down. Even the Hippocratic oath has been put aside as a mere suggestion of behaviors, rather than a profession's blueprint.

There must be those in the field who will stand firm in the belief that all human life is sacred, that our actions (and omissions) matter, and that our profession has a moral obligation to care and protect. If we fail to treat each patient as precious and of equal worth, if we fail to give optimal care to each patient that crosses our path, then the vulnerable, weak, and devalued patients could easily be victims of oppression and exploitation.[21] We have seen what the movement away from the Hippocratic oath could look like. One of the physicians who organized Hitler's medical euthanasia program, Dr. Karl Brandt, recognized that in order to get full support for implementation of the euthanasia program, the medical profession had to reject the Hippocratic oath. Starting in 1933, physicians took a new oath, which called on their service to the German state to be their primary loyalty. As Dr. Michael Franzblau, a Holocaust expert, commented, "Once you breach Hippocratic morality, only bad things can happen."[22] And in Charlie's recent book, he argues that when people who work in medicine do these bad things, they have an outsized impact on the culture at large.[23]

Nurses have the same ethical obligation to protect patients as physicians. Nurses aim at "the protection, promotion, and restoration of health and well-being; the prevention of illness and injury; and the alleviation of suffering, in the care of individuals, families, groups, communities, and populations."[24] There is no way to act in this way without a vision of the good—whether it is a religious vision or a secular one. As we saw in the previous chapter, there is simply no way for nurses to do their professional duty in light of their vision of the good without protecting their consciences. And those consciences must be protected when they offer their voice on health-care teams. And as important as the goals and values stated above are, the focus in this chapter has been on the role nurses play as experts in patient- and relationship-centered, whole-person care. And here we should remind ourselves that this is an absolutely essential insight of Trinitarian Christian theology. There is really no way to act for the good of the person without acting for their good *in relation-*

ships with others—but this is especially true in health care. Christian nurses with a Trinitarian vision should take their new place on medical teams confident that their vision is essential for creating a health-care system that genuinely centers on the holistic good of the patient.

A NOTE ABOUT RISKS FOR CHRISTIAN NURSES

Yes, we stand by the claim that nurses should be confident in doing this. But Alisha—as someone who has worn many different hats in health care (dietary aide, certified nursing assistant, registered nurse, family nurse practitioner, and professor)—understands the challenge that sometimes accompanies making her voice heard as a Christian. From making yourself vulnerable professionally by going around the traditional authority when a patient's life is at risk, to being left out of conversations and plans being made for a patient with whom you had the most contact, it can be frustrating and even professionally risky to act on one's behalf. One of the most frustrating things Alisha has encountered throughout the years is seeing a problem firsthand, having a solution to fix it, but not having a process in place for nurses to make change. Change most often happened from the top down and nurses, close to the bottom of the hierarchy, were often the last to hear of changes to protocols and procedures. They had little input on what care activities were actually part of the job requirement.

Alisha does bring some good news along with the bad, though. With the push toward morning huddles and bedside rounding, nurses are being invited to participate in care planning. While this is significant and a welcome change, it is nowhere near enough. Nurses need to not only insist on being in team meetings, but they need to have a formal space to speak up at those meetings. They should also be an equal voice on ethics committees and have a procedure in place for when an ethical dilemma arises. They need to have an avenue to make change at the organization level, as well as population health—lead health policy change, get involved in public health initiatives, and help transform health care from the bottom up. Nurses need to advocate for each patient, as well as their profession. Speak up. Push for change. Demand a seat at the table. And most importantly, make sure you are not forced to check your first principle—your Christian faith—at the door.

DISCUSSION QUESTIONS

1. This chapter emphasizes social determinants of health and claims that "by focusing on these sets of concerns moving forward, health-care systems and teams can help create physical and social environments that promote health and wellness for all." Do you agree? If so, what are some ways in which this can happen?
2. This chapter calls on nurses to play a greater role in shaping health-care change. Especially in light of what this chapter (and this book) has argued about the specific calling of nurses on health-care teams, what are some ways that nurses can get involved in leading the way to positive change?
3. Interprofessional collaboration is key to good patient care. Some hospitals try to promote this by having interdisciplinary rounds (with embedded chaplains, pharmacists, nurses, and social workers) or by having more shared workspaces to promote better relationships between team members. What are some other ways to promote this type of collaboration?

14

COVID-19 PANDEMIC AND BEYOND

To do what nobody else will do, in a way that nobody else can do, in spite of all we go through–that is to be a nurse.

– *Rawsi Williams*

It has become something close to a cliché to say that "everything will change" after the COVID-19 pandemic. In many cases these kinds of dramatic declarations are overstated, but for nursing we absolutely believe it to be true. There is simply no way that nursing can be the same after the pandemic and its impact on the profession. Nurses were the paradigmatic "front line workers" during the COVID-19 pandemic—and it was extremely fascinating (and often heartbreaking) to see the drama unfold in real time as we did the majority of our work on this book during the heart of this pandemic in the United States. In this, our final chapter, we explore the role nurses played during the pandemic, exploring both the good and the bad that occurred in what was an absolutely transformative year for nursing. We will then conclude the chapter and the book by reflecting about the implied coming changes for nursing, making one final call for Christian nurses to be clear and confident about their role in seeking out and achieving the changes necessary for a profession on the move.

THE CHALLENGES NURSES FACED DURING THE COVID-19 PANDEMIC

It was March 19, 2020, and Sonja Schwartzbach had had enough. A nurse in New Jersey at the height of one of the worst places in the US for the first wave of the pandemic, she realized the news media didn't really get how bad things were in hospitals. There was "such desperation" for her and her coworkers to get the story of their "war zones" out, she said, that she created an online document for her fellow nurses to share their stories. She had them do so anonymously, however, so that they could tell the whole truth about what was going on without losing their jobs. "There's also a history within nursing of retaliation," she said.[1]

The whole truth was nearly unbelievable. One veteran nurse wrote the following on Sonja's document: "Never seen anything like this. Protocols change minute to minute if there are any at all. I can no longer trust the CDC. For the first time in my career I am scared to go to work." Nurses were not only in the thick of what some called the "meat grinder" of the critical care units, but they were also primarily the ones who would try to comfort the dying, aid those who were recovering, and accompany those with uncertain futures. One nurse on the frontlines told her story to Charlie this way:

> During the first week of COVID-19 I couldn't have imagined seeing the light at the end of the tunnel for health-care workers or patients. It was chaotic, terrifying, confusing, etc. It was just you and coronavirus in a room, door sealed shut. I wrapped more body bags in a week than I did in my entire nursing career. Families begging for photos or FaceTimes with their deceased family member as their "last goodbye." Very traumatic. Insane to even think about going into a room and taking a photo or FaceTiming with a dead person and that being someone's last goodbye. My first intubated COVID

> patient that week broke my heart by asking me if she was going to die, while also apologizing for possibly infecting me with the virus. I thought those might be her last words. To be honest, I didn't know—so we both cried. I was scared for her and for me, she was scared for her and for me too. Today she squeezed my hand for the first time in 8 weeks. And today I look forward to going to work for the first time in weeks to see her progress as she starts to make a FULL recovery (shout-out to my SICU [surgical intensive care unit] team!).[2]

A powerful storytelling project—the result of a partnership of "Dear World" and the American Association of Critical Care Nurses—has helped tell the story of nurses during the pandemic far and wide.[3] "Everyone mostly dies," one nurse said. "In the ICU I've seen very few people walk out." Many nurses were performing functions for which they are were not trained. One charge nurse reflected on his time leading a team of redeployed nurses for his COVID-19 ICU—nurses who weren't used to seeing the sickness of a normal ICU, much less one during the height of a new and frightening pandemic. After his first shift, during which three patients died, he called his girlfriend in the car crying and reflecting the utter chaos he had just experienced. When he got home his roommate reminded him of the John Wayne quote "Courage is being scared to death, but saddling up anyway."

And there was plenty of reason to be scared to death. Not just for fear of their patients' lives, but their own lives as well. One of the key reveals of Sonja's project was just how poor the equipment so many nurses were working with in the early stages of the pandemic. The lack of personal protective equipment (PPE) is by now a well-worn part of the story of the early pandemic, but fewer know the extreme lengths nurses went to in order to care for patients. "We are being called to jeopardize our own health and safety to treat our community," one California nurse said. "We live in the richest country in the world and yet we don't have the tools to perform our job safely." They were asked to keep the same surgical mask on for their entire shift and could only get an N95 mask in certain situations. One Pennsylvania nurse wrote, "We actually got an email saying not to remove gloves when in a room if they get soiled, but to use sanitizer on the gloves!"[4]

HOW NURSES RESPONDED

Despite all of this, most nurses—many already overworked in a traditional setting—were something close to heroic in standing strong on the front lines of the fight against the pandemic. And good thing, too, because nurses as usual brought important expertise to bear that was essential for the fight. Much of this involved direct care to patients, particularly in the ICU, but nurses were also involved in organizing the new pandemic workforces, advising governments, leading research teams, and coordinating public health responses.[5] Experienced critical care nurses, for instance, were largely responsible for creating an ad hoc process in which massive numbers of general nurses, retired nurses, and even undergraduate nursing students were trained on the fly to do tasks with which they were unfamiliar. While physicians, also working the frontlines, were the main ones on news programs and making headlines in Washington, DC, nurses were working behind the scenes by advising local governments, cutting through the noise and using their on-the-ground expertise to carefully address what was often very localized and specific contexts.

But beyond specific, technical expertise is the vocation or calling of nurses to offer care of the whole person. Never was this calling to care for vulnerable patients in a holistic way more important than during the pandemic. Nurses not only worked with the medical team to treat and stabilize patients, they were at the very center of most patients' recoveries. With physical distancing and isolation measures in place, nurses were often the primary source of human contact for these patients—contact that was absolutely essential for their return to health. They were also forced to get creative in thinking about the good of their patients in relationship with others. The family-centered care they offered often involved phone or the internet, setting up conversations with loved ones "sometimes just before endotracheal intubation and mechanical ventilation from which many will not recover."[6] The creation of a "virtual bedside," though not unknown before the pandemic, was something countless families benefited from because of the creative work of nurses.

At a time when so much of the health-care process was medicalized—and the "care" part seeming to go by the wayside in many circumstances—nurses of the pandemic were beacons of humanity and human dignity. We asked several nurses in our circles what they learned most from the pandemic and it was striking how many responses focused on this general topic. Here are just a few:

> I learned to understand that the need to be seen as *imago Dei* is a part of the healing process. That people are not a liability or a malpractice suit.

> We are dealing now with the aftereffects of one year of masking/PPE and when dealing with patients as human beings, caring for them, being empathetic and in nursing them, we are pulling our masks down, because they need to see us smile. They need to feel comforted by our faces. They need to feel our ungloved hand, especially as they have been isolated from family.

> I have learned that nursing fundamentals (like, literally what you learned in your first fundamentals class) is what mattered most in keeping (my elderly) people alive through this.

There is just something so beautiful about these insights. And they remind us of Annella's description in chapter 9 of her patient "Rebecca" who she was caring for in a nursing home during the pandemic:

> Changing patients is like a choreographed dance. You gather your supplies, you put the bed up high, and you do everything in halves—you strip half of the bed, roll them away from you, tuck everything tight under them, roll them back to you, and the same with the diapers. Roll, roll, roll. It takes so much out of them, when they have so little energy to spare that it's exhausting. But I got her cleaned up, dry, we washed her face, put cream on her arms and legs, got fresh sheets on, and I got her covered up with fresh sheets and a blanket. Pretty soon Rebecca was as snug as a bug in a rug, fast asleep with a very different look on her face.

This book has made it clear that this kind of focus on the full humanity of the patient—and not just on mitigating an isolated and medicalized view of disease—is at the heart of the call to be a nurse. The focus on human touch, clean and cared for skin, and the feel of fresh sheets are, by themselves, all beautiful examples of such care. And imagining the changing an adult patient's undergarments as a kind of dance is almost stunning in its counter-cultural humanity. But this is how the majority of nurses responded during the pandemic: they fought for, cared for, and honored the full humanity of their patients under some of the most difficult circumstances imaginable.

STRESSORS DRAMATICALLY INCREASED

Perhaps the worst thing to come out of the pandemic for nurses and nursing is the incredible stressors and burnout so many experienced. The amount of death they have witnessed; the amount of grief they have seen in families (and experienced themselves); the ridiculous conditions in which they had to perform; all of these have taken their toll on nurses during the pandemic. For many newer nurses, it was especially traumatic as they had never experienced anything remotely like it before. For some older nurses, it was something akin to the straw breaking the camel's back. In addition to work weeks and weeks without a break, nurses were also "the go-to person for family and friends at work and home: there is no 'off' button."[7] Couple this with nurses self-isolating at home, distanced from the physical touch and personal presence that normally fills their emotional and spiritual cups, and you have a recipe for major trauma. And that trauma is having predictable results, with nurses deciding to leave the profession in large numbers.[8]

Though it varies from region to region, there was a nursing shortage in the United States even before the pandemic.[9] An aging population, along with an aging nursing workforce, accounted for a large portion of the problem. Given that significant percentages of nurses are women of childbearing age, inadequate opportunities and structures for combining nursing with being a mother have also contributed to the shortage and new mothers often leave the nursing workforce and then choose jobs with more flexibility down the road. Further, again even before the pandemic, there was intense pressure on nurses especially from profit-centered hospitals and clinics doing the absolute minimum when it came to nurse staffing. One nurse, who formerly worked as a charge nurse, told Charlie about putting together the spreadsheet laying out how many patients and staff would be on the floor at a given time. She was taught to keep staffing at the minimal amount required for the current census. If they had one more nurse than was deemed "required," she would "flex" one nurse home without pay for the rest of the shift. It was a difficult balancing act, because they would also have to predict how many patients would be admitted. It was not uncommon that she would send staff home early and the floor would later get slammed with admissions. And she would be reprimanded if they operated with "extra" staff for even a couple hours.

These kinds of structures lead to nurse/patient ratios that are simply untenable and nurses trained in one specific area being forced to do the jobs of several other disciplines. "We are expected to play all these roles, chart in real time, keep our patients alive, all while striving to achieve perfect satisfaction scores on our surveys," the former charge nurse said. "We need to do this in 12 hours, which seems like a lot, but can go by so quickly before you realize that you forgot to go to the bathroom or eat for the entire shift."[10] In part due to these structures and expectations, non-bedside jobs in nursing are becoming extremely competitive as many nurses leave the stress of directly caring for patients in beds without the proper resources. Add the stressors and trauma of the pandemic and you've got a recipe for a major staffing and resource problem—again, as the population at large continues to age and more beds and bedside staff are needed. And younger nurses—the ones we might expect to fill that future gap—are at particular risk for leaving.[11] They've been thrown into the mess of the pandemic without the professional, mental, or (often) spiritual resources to cope. Alisha has seen this as a graduate nursing professor. She asks each student why they decided to return to school to become a nurse practitioner. While many say they had always planned on doing so, or they felt a calling, there is a large number of students who say they are burned out working in a hospital setting and decided to return to school for a "new career."

THE FUTURE

This is a disastrous situation. Just as the population is aging—and in clear need of many more bedside nurses—we are losing many of the bedside nurses we already had, including a disproportionate percentage of the younger ones. We discussed elsewhere in this book how bad the "care left undone" crisis already is—and what this will likely mean into the future (especially for older populations with dementia and/or in nursing home) is, frankly, scary to think about. If we are to avoid profound cases of neglect, the slouch toward assisted suicide, or the impersonal care that comes from robots, we simply must find a way to encourage nurses to stay by the bedside and recruit more young people to become nurses in the future.

And this process begins with nurses themselves aggressively demanding change. We discussed this in the previous chapter, but especially in a post-pandemic health-care moment already full of ferment and creative possibility this change can look even more realistic. The old view of the role of nurses—expressed well by the phrase "you are only a number here and I can have someone else fill your job in an instant"[12]—is not long for this world. As chapter 13 demonstrated, nurses have an essential role on health-care teams and nurses must advocate for themselves for their rightful place on such teams. And not only that, but nurses must advocate for appropriate staffing and concern for their mental/psychological health as well. As one nurse shared:

> Employers must realize we aren't machines and must take care of our mental health needs too. We can't work for pay and benefits without a reprieve from the losses so many experienced in ICU and COVID units. Even those of us in surgical centers felt the pressure to work constantly. Pizza isn't a remedy but our bosses may think it is. We need flexibility instead of constant stress of visitor restrictions and lonely patients who are getting delirious from the lack of stimulation. We need to stop stuffing down our feelings and be real—no more Mr. Nice Guy just because the unit is shorthanded and the new grads don't have a real preceptor experience. No more yard signs saying "Heroes Work Here." Develop some real

> help for those suffering from the work-related stress instead of sending out daily texts begging us to pick up another shift for a bonus. My coworkers are tired from the constant stress. I'm tired of employers not responding to my job apps. There's a lack of communication in a system that thrives on communication. Surgical centers need to run on real-time staffing, not filling up the surgery schedule and wonder why they don't have enough critical care nurses to receive the post op patients . . . [and] need to check on the mental health of their nurses before they burn out.

Happily, there does seem to be some evidence that, finally, real attention is being paid to the mental health needs of health-care workers.[13]

Yet mental health is very much related to spiritual health. And it is with this topic we'd like to conclude our book on a Christian bioethical vision for nurses. Though for some folks nursing is little more than a job which pays the bills, for a faithful Christian it is part of his broader vocation and broader commitment to live out the gospel of Jesus Christ. An active life of prayer and other spiritual practices (in community with other Christians, and other Christian nurses, if possible) is something close to necessary to do this job well as a Christian. For it is in relationship with God and others that Christians refill our spiritual cups and remind ourselves of why we do what we do. Recall the Sisters of Mercy focusing on self-care as an essential part of the nurse's vocation. Loving oneself—one's *whole* self—is something that Christ teaches us is intimately connected to loving one's neighbor. And this is especially true if this neighbor is a vulnerable patient, lying prone on a hospital bed, requiring your care in order to thrive, survive, or even live their last few weeks or days of life with dignity.

Not everyone is fortunate enough to have a profession that is so clearly connected to the gospel of Jesus Christ. While nearly all work is dignified and can be ordered to the glory of God, some is so obviously connected to seeing the face of Christ in the vulnerable and marginalized that it pulls the believer even closer to the goal of loving God with her whole heart, soul, mind, and strength. Some professions help the believer refuse a false distinction between "my life as a Christian" on the one hand and "my work life" on the other. Nursing is clearly one of these professions and the Christian nurse should acknowledge this especially privileged position. She is constantly surrounded by people who bear the face of Christ in a special way, a way which calls the Christian out of herself to other-centered love.

Especially in light of the coming crisis in health-care resources, if we are going to meet the health-care needs of the developed West in the future it is overwhelmingly likely that Christian nurses will be at the center of doing so. In living out the gospel in this context, Christian nurses not only find an important way to fulfill their own religious and spiritual duties on the level of the individual, but also their social duties to serve the broader culture and needs of their local communities. If we are to avoid the slouch toward euthanasia and robots—if we are to avoid the neglect that comes from treating vulnerable people as throwaway populations—Christian nurses will need to be at the heart of that resistance. (This, as we mentioned earlier in the book, will be especially true in nursing homes and the field of geriatrics.) And though all of this entails doing very hard work—work that is not without risk, as Alisha reminded us in the previous chapter—it is the kind of authentic work that fulfills one at the deepest levels of who they are. It also involves precisely the kind of other-centered love that opens non-believers to the faith. Authentic Christian love is one of the most important ways that people become attracted to the gospel from which it comes.

At our most hopeful, Charlie and Alisha can imagine the creation of a virtuous cycle in which more and more people are drawn to be Christian nurses as a means of both (1) loving God, self, and neighbor and (2) meeting the cultural needs of the moment and of the (near) future. In doing so, especially if they insist on performing their vocation in line with the religious and spiritual commitments that brought them to the profession in the first place, they connect themselves to other Christian nurses who have done similar kinds of work throughout the centuries.[14]

Our forebearers blazed the paths we are privileged to walk today. Let us not squander the gifts we have been given by God and (in a related story) by those who have gone before us by fearfully burying them in the ground. Rather, let the light of Christian nurses shine before the broader culture, bearing fruit for Christ Jesus, the center of all that we are and all that we do.

DISCUSSION QUESTIONS

1. The COVID-19 pandemic brought with it a steep learning curve for all members of the health-care team. What did we learn in the process? What does it mean for providing health care going forward (even when the COVID-19 pandemic wanes and conditions return to a more normal state)?
2. One of the major problems of the COVID-19 pandemic is that medical teams and institutions were not prepared. What sorts of things do we need to have in place before another pandemic arrives?
3. This book has tried to offer a vision of nursing as a vocation that honors God, the nurse, the patient, and the community in which the care is being given. What are some of the key concepts that you took from this book? And how will these concepts guide your nursing care moving forward?

NOTES

Introduction

1. "Nursing and Midwifery," World Health Organization, https://www.who.int/hrh/nursing_midwifery/en/.

2. Harriet Sherwood, "Religion: Why Faith Is Becoming More and More Popular," *The Guardian*, August 27, 2018, https://www.theguardian.com/news/2018/aug/27/religion-why-is-faith-growing-and-what-happens-next.

3. "NP Fact Sheet," American Association of Nurse Practitioners, 2020, https://www.aanp.org/about/all-about-nps/np-fact-sheet#:~:text=There%20are%20more%20than%20290%2C000,NPs)%20licensed%20in%20the%20U.S.&text=More%20than%2028%2C700%20new%20NPs,academic%20programs%20in%202017%E2%80%932018.

4. "Nursing Fact Sheet," American Association of Colleges of Nursing, April 1, 2019, https://www.aacnnursing.org/News-Information/Fact-Sheets/Nursing-Fact-Sheet#:~:text=Nursing%20is%20the%20nation's%20largest,84.5%25%20are%20employed%20in%20nursing.&text=The%20federal%20government%20projects%20that,each%20year%20from%202016%2D2026.

5. And very often the context matters quite a bit. For instance, for Black Americans who are "nones" (people who don't identify with any religious faith), a whopping 90 percent still believe in God or other higher power. And 36 percent of that 90 percent still believe

in the God of the Bible. https://www.pewresearch.org/fact-tank/2021/03/17/nine-in-ten-black-nones-believe-in-god-but-fewer-pray-or-attend-services/.

6. "Religion in America: U.S. Religious Data, Demographics and Statistics," Pew Research Center's Religion and Public Life Project, Pew Research Center, September 19, 2018, https://www.pewforum.org/religious-landscape-study/.

7. "Religion in America: Religious Nones," Pew Research Center's Religion and Public Life Project, Pew Research Center, September 19, 2018, https://www.pewforum.org/religious-landscape-study/religious-tradition/unaffiliated-religious-nones/#demographic-information.

8. Laura Santhanam, "New Study Shows 1 in 6 U.S. Health Care Workers Are Immigrants," *PBS*, December 5, 2018, https://www.pbs.org/newshour/health/new-study-shows-1-in-6-u-s-health-care-workers-are-immigrants.

9. Nathalie Robles, "Why Filipino Nurses Are a Huge Presence in U.S. Health Care," *INQUIRER.NET*, May 3, 2019, https://usa.inquirer.net/28681/why-filipino-nurses-are-a-huge-presence-in-u-s-health-care.

10. Kris Haldeman, "What's Unique in Christian Caring?," *Journal of Christian Nursing* 23, no. 3 (Summer 2006): 20–21, https://doi.org/10.1097/00005217-200608000-00007.

11. For most on this history, see Charles Curran, "The Catholic Moral Tradition in Bioethics" in *The Story of Bioethics: From Seminal Works to Contemporary Explorations* (Washington, DC: Georgetown University Press, 2003), 113–30.

Chapter 1

1. Mary C. Sullivan, ed., *The Friendship of Florence Nightingale and Mary Clare Moore* (Philadelphia: University of Pennsylvania Press, 1999).

2. Much of what we say in this section comes from that section of his book. Charles C. Camosy, *Losing Our Dignity: How Secularized*

Medicine Is Undermining Fundamental Human Equality (Hyde Park, NY: New City Press, 2021). Reprinted by permission.

3. Rodney Stark, *The Rise of Christianity: A Sociologist Reconsiders History* (Princeton, NJ: Princeton University Press, 1996).

4. J. J. Walsh, "Hospitals," in *The Catholic Encyclopedia* (New York: Robert Appleton Company, 1910), retrieved from New Advent, http://www.newadvent.org/cathen/07480a.htm.

5. Roy Porter, *The Greatest Benefit to Mankind: A Medical History of Humanity from Antiquity to the Present* (New York; London: Harper Collins, 1997), 112.

6. Andrew T. Crislip, *From Monastery to Hospital: Christian Monasticism and the Transformation of Health Care in Late Antiquity* (Ann Arbor: University of Michigan Press, 2005).

7. Walsh, "Hospitals."

8. "Our History," Filles Du St. Esprit, 2017, https://www.fillesstesprit.org/site/english/716.html.

9. Tim McHugh, "Expanding Women's Rural Medical Work in Early Modern Brittany: The Daughters of the Holy Spirit," *Journal of the History of Medicine and Allied Sciences* 67, no. 3 (July 2012): 428–56, https://doi-org.avoserv2.library.fordham.edu/10.1093/jhmas/jrr032.

10. Suzie Farren, "The Sister Nurses," *Journal of the Catholic Health Association of the United States* (March/April 2003), https://www.chausa.org/publications/health-progress/article/march-april-2003/the-sister-nurses.

11. "Our History," Daughters of the Holy Spirit, USA Province, (2018) https://daughtersoftheholyspirit.org/our-history/.

12. Therese Meehan, "Great Tenderness in All Things," *Careful Nursing: Philosophy and Professional Practice Model* (July 2016), https://www.carefulnursing.ie/go/blog/2016-07/great-tenderness-in-all-things.

13. Meehan, "Great Tenderness."

14. For a full list and for more details, see https://www.chausa.org/docs/default-source/general-files/contemporary_nursing_practice_model-pdf.pdf?sfvrsn=0.

15. Sullivan, *Friendship*, 5.

16. Sullivan, *Friendship*, 8.

17. Therese Meehan, "Spirituality and Spiritual Care from a Careful Nursing Perspective," *Journal of Nursing Management* (2012), http://citeseerx.ist.psu.edu/viewdoc/download?doi=10.1.1.1008.6851&rep=rep1&type=pdf.

18. Therese Meehan, "Careful Nursing: A Model for Contemporary Nursing Practice," *Journal of Advanced Nursing* 21, no. 19 (May 30, 2003): 99–107, https://www.chausa.org/docs/default-source/general-files/contemporary_nursing_practice_model-pdf.pdf?sfvrsn=0.

19. Sullivan, *Friendship*, 14.

20. Sullivan, *Friendship*, 18.

21. Sullivan, *Friendship*, 30.

22. Sullivan, *Friendship*, 21.

23. Sullivan, *Friendship*, 26.

24. Sullivan, *Friendship*, 43.

25. Sullivan, *Friendship*, 181.

26. Sullivan, *Friendship*, 183.

27. Mary P. Kelly, "Hospital Nuns: From the Civil War to Today," *Irish America*, September 18, 2018, https://irishamerica.com/2013/08/hospital-nuns-from-the-civil-war-to-today/.

28. Ann Rodgers, "Union's Top Military Nurses Were Nuns," *Pittsburgh Post-Gazette*, June 30, 2013, https://www.post-gazette.com/news/state/2013/06/30/Union-s-top-military-nurses-were-nuns/stories/201306300137.

29. B. M. Wall, "Definite Lines of Influence: Catholic Sisters and Nurse Training Schools, 1890-1920," *Nursing Research* 50, no. 5 (September/October 2001): 314–21, https://pubmed.ncbi.nlm.nih.gov/11570717/.

30. Indeed, Charlie recently gave a talk at Mercy College of Health Sciences in Des Moines, Iowa, which was founded as a nursing school by the Sisters of Mercy in 1899. Charlie is deeply indebted to conversations he had there, especially with Bo Bonner, for many ideas which shaped his contributions to this book.

31. Emma Green, "Nuns vs. the Coronavirus," *The Atlantic*, May 3,

2020, https://www.theatlantic.com/politics/archive/2020/05/coronavirus-nursing-home-deaths/611053/.

Chapter 2

1. Harold G. Koenig, "Religion and Medicine I: Historical Background and Reasons for Separation," *The International Journal of Psychiatry in Medicine* 30, no. 4 (December 2000): 385–98, http://citeseerx.ist.psu.edu/viewdoc/download?doi=10.1.1.521.9908&rep=rep1&type=pdf.

2. Michael J. Pritchard, "Is It Time to Re-Examine the Doctor-Nurse Relationship since the Introduction of the Independent Nurse Prescriber?," *Australian Journal of Advanced Nursing* 35 (2017): 31, https://www.ajan.com.au/archive/Vol35/Issue2/4Pritchard.pdf.

3. Pritchard, "Time to Re-Examine?," 31.

4. J. McGregor Robertson, *The Physician* (London: Gresham Publishing, 1902).

5. Dorothy Jones, "Are We Abandoning Nursing as a Discipline?," *Clinical Nurse Specialist* 19, no. 6 (2005): 275–77, https://www.nursingcenter.com/journalarticle?Article_ID=613974&Journal_ID=54033&Issue_ID=613973.

6. Kathy Quan, "In the Year of the Nurse, Four Million Nurses Have a Voice and Need to Take a Stand," *Nursing CE* (blog), January 22, 2020, https://www.nursingce.com/blog/the-year-of-the-nurse/.

7. Bushra Mushtaq and Javaid Ahmad Mir, "Nursing as Academic Discipline and a Profession," *JOJ Nursing and Healthcare* 8, no. 1 (May 2018), https://juniperpublishers.com/jojnhc/pdf/JOJNHC.MS.ID.555730.pdf.

8. Mushtaq and Mir, "Nursing."

9. Jones, "Abandoning Nursing?"

10. "The Critical Role of a Nurse: Bridging the Gap between Art & Science," *The Sentinel Blog*, January 8, 2018, http://www.css.edu/the-sentinel-blog/the-critical-role-of-a-nurse-bridging-the-gap-between-art-and-science.html.

11. "Critical Role of a Nurse."

12. Quoted in Ginny Roth, "Nurses: The Heart of Healing," *Circulating Now*, May 6, 2014, https://circulatingnow.nlm.nih.gov/2014/05/06/nurses-the-heart-of-healing/.

13. "Critical Role of a Nurse."

14. Sheria Grice Robinson, "True Presence: Practicing the Art of Nursing," *Nursing* 44, no. 4 (April 2014): 44–45, https://doi.org/10.1097/01.nurse.0000444533.58704.e5.

15. Carrie Dameron, "What Is the Essence of Christian Nursing?," *Journal of Christian Nursing* 27, no. 4 (October–December 2010): 285, https://journals.lww.com/journalofchristiannursing/Citation/2010/12000/What_Is_the_Essence_of_Christian_Nursing_.3.aspx.

16. Mary Elizabeth O'Brien, *Spirituality in Nursing: Standing on Holy Ground*, 6th ed. (Burlington, MA: Jones & Bartlett Learning, 2018), 25.

17. Suyin Haynes, "How Florence Nightingale Paved the Way for the Heroic Work of Nurses Today," *Time Magazine*, May 12, 2020, https://time.com/5835150/florence-nightingale-legacy-nurses/.

18. O'Brien, *Spirituality in Nursing*, 33.

19. Peter J. Levin, "Bold Vision: Catholic Sisters and the Creation of American Hospitals," *Journal of Community Health* 36 (2011): 343–47, https://link.springer.com/article/10.1007/s10900-011-9401-7.

20. Mathew H. Gendle, "The Problem of Dualism in Modern Western Medicine," *Mens Sana Monographs* 14, no. 1 (2016): 141–51, https://www.ncbi.nlm.nih.gov/pmc/articles/PMC5179613/.

21. Judith Allen Shelly, *Called to Care: A Christian Worldview for Nursing* (Downers Grove, IL: IVP Academic, 2006).

22. "What Is Holistic Nursing?" *Northeastern State University Online Nursing*, March 6, 2019, https://nursingonline.nsuok.edu/articles/rnbsn/what-is-holistic-nursing.aspx.

23. Shelly, *Called to Care*, 16.

24. Monya De, "Towards Defining Paternalism in Medicine," *The Virtual Mentor* 6, no. 2 (2004): 55–57, https://journalofethics.ama-assn.org/article/towards-defining-paternalism-medicine/2004-02.

25. De, "Paternalism in Medicine."

26. Brian C. Drolet and Candace L. White, "Selective Paternalism,"

The Virtual Mentor 14, no. 7 (2012): 582–88, https://journalofethics.ama-assn.org/article/selective-paternalism/2012-07.

27. Christina Gresh, "The Caring Art of Nursing," *NursingCenter Blog*, May 28, 2019, https://www.nursingcenter.com/ncblog/may-2019/the-caring-art-of-nursing.

28. "Code of Ethics for Nurses with Interpretive Statements," *American Nurses Association*, 2015, https://www.nursingworld.org/practice-policy/nursing-excellence/ethics/code-of-ethics-for-nurses/coe-view-only/.

29. Arlene Keeling, "Historical Perspectives on an Expanded Role for Nursing," *OJIN: The Online Journal of Issues in Nursing* 20, no. 2 (May 31, 2015), http://ojin.nursingworld.org/MainMenuCategories/ANAMarketplace/ANAPeriodicals/OJIN/TableofContents/Vol-20-2015/No2-May-2015/Historical-Perspectives-Expanded-Role-Nursing.html.

30. Hannah Dellabella, "50 Years of the Nurse Practitioner Profession," *Clinical Advisor*, November 10, 2015, https://www.clinicaladvisor.com/home/web-exclusives/50-years-of-the-nurse-practitioner-profession/.

31. "Year of the Nurse and the Midwife 2020," World Health Organization, https://www.who.int/campaigns/year-of-the-nurse-and-the-midwife-2020.

32. "The Future of Nursing: Leading Change, Advancing Health," Institute of Medicine (US) Committee on the Robert Wood Johnson Foundation Initiative on the Future of Nursing, at the Institute of Medicine (Washington, DC: National Academies Press, 2011).

Chapter 3

1. Kristin Collier, "Spirituality and Religion in Medicine—Why Should You Care?," *MD UM Gen Med Grand Rounds*, August 21, 2020, https://medicine.umich.edu/dept/intmed/education-training/medicine-grand-rounds.

2. Michael J. Balboni and Tracy A. Balboni, *Hostility to Hospitality:*

Spirituality and Professional Socialization within Medicine (New York: Oxford University Press, 2019), 100.

3. Daniel Peterson, "Galileo: Science vs. Religion or Truth vs. Fiction?," *Deseret News*, July 22, 2020, https://www.deseret.com/faith/2020/7/22/21321364/daniel-peterson-galileo-galilei-science-vs-religion-or-truth-vs-fiction.

4. Maurice A. Finocchiaro, ed., *The Galileo Affair: A Documentary History* (Berkeley: University of California Press, 1989), 67–69.

5. Kenneth Briggs, "Scholars Are Still Embattled Over the Case of Galileo," *The New York Times*, April 28, 1981, https://www.nytimes.com/1981/04/28/science/scholars-are-still-embattled-over-the-case-of-galileo-madisonwisc.html.

6. Viktor Blåsjö, "Intellectual Mathematics," *Intellectual Mathematics* (blog), January 18, 2019, http://intellectualmathematics.com/blog/galileos-theory-of-tides/.

7. Udo Schuklenk, "Professionalism Eliminates Religion as a Proper Tool for Doctors Rendering Advice to Patients," *Journal of Medical Ethics* 45, no. 11 (2019): 713.

8. Rachel Browne, "Medical Schools Should Deny Applicants Who Object to Provide Abortion, Assisted Death: Bioethicist," *Global News*, November 23, 2019, https://globalnews.ca/news/6183548/medical-school-applicants-abortion-assisted-death-conscientious-objectors/.

9. Oscar Riddle, *Biographical Memoir of Charles Benedict Davenport 1866–1944* (National Academy of Sciences, 1947), www.nasonline.org/publications/biographical-memoirs/memoir-pdfs/davenport-charles.pdf.

10. Adam Cohen, "Harvard's Eugenics Era," *Harvard Magazine*, (2016), https://harvardmagazine.com/2016/03/harvards-eugenics-era.

11. M. Berghs, B. Dierckx de Casterlé, and C. Gastmans, "Nursing, Obedience, and Complicity with Eugenics: A Contextual Interpretation of Nursing Morality at the Turn of the Twentieth Century," *Journal of Medical Ethics* 32, no. 2 (2006): 117–22, https://doi.org/10.1136/jme.2004.011171.

12. For some details about US practices see Terry Gross, interview

with Adam Cohen, "The Supreme Court Ruling That Led to 70,000 Forced Sterilizations," *NPR's Fresh Air*, podcast audio, March 7, 2016, https://www.npr.org/sections/health-shots/2016/03/07/469478098/the-supreme-court-ruling-that-led-to-70-000-forced-sterilizations.

13. Audrey Farla, "The Revival of Raced-Based Medicine: Eugenics, Religion, and the Black Experience," review of *Medical Stigmata*, by K. A. Johnson, Marginalia, *Los Angeles Review of Books*, October 18, 2019, https://marginalia.lareviewofbooks.org/revival-of-raced-based-medicine-eugenics-religion-and-the-black-experience/.

14. Pope Pius XI, *Casti Connubii*, Vatican website, December 31, 1930, https://w2.vatican.va/content/pius-xi/en/encyclicals/documents/hf_p-xi_enc_19301231_casti-connubii.html.

15. Charles McDaniel, "A Model for Christian Engagement in the Age of Consumer Eugenics" (American Eugenics Society Conference, Baylor University, 2018), https://www.stthomas.edu/media/catholicstudies/center/ryan/conferences/2018-stpaul/McDanielRyanConferencePaper6718.pdf.

16. Richard J. Evans, *The Third Reich at War* (New York: Penguin, 2009), 100.

17. Wolfgang Neugebauer, "The Nazi Mass Murder of the Intellectually and the Physically Disabled and the Resistance of Sister Anna Bertha Königsegg," Lecture, Documentation Archive of the Austrian Resistance, Goldegg Castle, November 12, 1998, https://www.doew.at/cms/download/d7kv5/wn_koenigsegg.pdf?fbclid=IwAR3-S8LENudyrMv7QvrIrhDKZZeMpyLyoxwXkSw_MrdoL_ub-XXpE5WcaYA.

Chapter 4

1. For a nice and accessible argument along these lines, see Terrence W. Tilley, *Faith: What It Is and What It Isn't* (Maryknoll, NY: Orbis Books, 2010).

2. To name just one of several examples, we take much of the insight below from Congregation for the Doctrine of the Faith, *Samaritanus Bonus: On the Care of Persons in the Critical and Terminal Phases of Life*, Encyclical Letter, Vatican website, November 21, 1964, http://

www.vatican.va/roman_curia/congregations/cfaith/documents/rc_con_cfaith_doc_20200714_samaritanus-bonus_en.html.

3. Daniel Horan, "Embracing Sister Death: The Fraternal Worldview of Francis of Assisi as a Source for Christian Eschatological Hope," *The Other Journal* 14 (2009), https://theotherjournal.com/2009/01/20/embracing-sister-death-the-fraternal-worldview-of-francis-of-assisi-as-a-source-for-christian-eschatological-hope/.

4. Adolf von Harnack, *The Expansion of Christianity in the First Three Centuries, Volume 1* (California: Putnam, 1904).

5. American Medical Association, "Physician Assisted Suicide," in *AMA Principles of Medical Ethics: I, II, IV, VI, VIII, IX*, https://www.ama-assn.org/delivering-care/ethics/physician-assisted-suicide.

6. Richard M. Doerflinger, "The Effect of Legalizing Assisted Suicide on Palliative Care and Suicide Rates: A Response to Compassion and Choices," *Charlotte Lozier Institute: On Point* 13 (2017), https://lozierinstitute.org/the-effect-of-legalizing-assisted-suicide-on-palliative-care-and-suicide-rates/.

7. John F. Kilner, "The Bible, Ethics, and Health Care: Theological Foundations for a Christian Perspective on Health Care," https://www.wheaton.edu/media/migrated-images-amp-files/media/files/centers-and-institutes/cace/booklets/BibleEthicsHealthcare.pdf.

8. Christian Medical and Dental Associations, "Biblical Model for Medical Ethics," *CMDA Ethics Statements*, 2018, https://cmda.org/wp-content/uploads/2018/04/Biblical-Model-with-References.pdf.

9. Kilner, "Bible, Ethics, and Health Care."

Chapter 5

1. Mark Mercurio, "The Aftermath of Baby Doe and the Evolution of Newborn Intensive Care," *Georgia State University Law Review* 25, no. 4 (2012): 1–31, https://readingroom.law.gsu.edu/cgi/viewcontent.cgi?article=2389&context=gsulr.

2. Leo Alexander, "Medical Science under Dictatorship," *The New England Journal of Medicine* (July 14, 1949): 39–47.

3. Brian Clowes, "Is Nazi Euthanasia Resurfacing in the U.S.?," *Hu-*

man Life International, July 24, 2020, https://www.hli.org/resources/nazi-euthanasia/.

4. Anne Scott, Clare Harvey, Heike Felzmann, Riitta Suhonen, Monika Habermann, Kristin Halvorsen, Karin Christiansen, Luisa Toffoli, and Evridiki Papastavrou, "Resource Allocation and Rationing in Nursing Care: A Discussion Paper," *Nursing Ethics* 26, no. 5 (2019): 1528–39, https://journals.sagepub.com/doi/full/10.1177/0969733018759831.

5. B. J. Kalisch, G. Landstrom, and A. Hinshaw, "Missed Nursing Care: A Concept Analysis," *Journal of Advanced Nursing* 67, no. 7 (2009): 1509–17.

6. N. L. Falk and E. S. Chong, "Beyond the Bedside: Nurses, a Critical Force in the Macroallocation of Resources," *OJIN: The Online Journal of Issues in Nursing* 13, no. 2 (2008), http://ojin.nursingworld.org/MainMenuCategories/ANAMarketplace/ANAPeriodicals/OJIN/TableofContents/vol132008/No2May08/ArticlePreviousTopic/MacroallocationofResources.html.

7. Scott, Harvey, Felzmann, Suhonen, Habermann, Halvorsen, Christiansen, Toffoli, and Papastavrou, "Resource Allocation and Rationing in Nursing Care."

8. Meina Lee and Elizabeth Geelhoed, "Teaching Resource Allocation—And Why It Matters," *AMA Journal of Ethics* 13, no. 4 (2011): 224–27, https://journalofethics.ama-assn.org/article/teaching-resource-allocation-and-why-it-matters/2011-04.

9. Lee and Geelhoed, "Teaching Resource Allocation."

10. Michael White, "The End at the Beginning," *The Ochsner Journal* 11, no. 4 (2011): 309–16, https://www.ncbi.nlm.nih.gov/pmc/articles/PMC3241062/.

11. Jeff Lyon, "The Death of Baby Doe," *The Chicago Tribune*, February 10, 1985, https://www.chicagotribune.com/news/ct-xpm-1985-02-10-8501080761-story.html.

12. Abigail Lawlis Kuzma, "The Legislative Response to Infant Doe," *Indiana Law Journal* 59, no. 3 (1984): 378–416, https://www.repository.law.indiana.edu/cgi/viewcontent.cgi?article=2208&context=ilj.

13. Lyon, "Death of Baby Doe."

14. Mercurio, "Aftermath of Baby Doe."

15. Kuzma, "Legislative Response."

16. Kuzma, "Legislative Response."

17. "Baby Doe Case: A Life Not Worth Living?" *Right To Life Michigan*, n.d., https://rtl.org/infanticide/baby-doe-case/.

18. Lyon, "Death of Baby Doe."

19. Lyon, "Death of Baby Doe."

20. Mercurio, "Aftermath of Baby Doe."

21. Mercurio, "Aftermath of Baby Doe."

22. Kuzma, "Legislative Response."

23. Kuzma, "Legislative Response."

24. Katherine Kortsmit et al., "Abortion Surveillance - United States, 2018," *Morbidity and Mortality Weekly Report Surveillance Summaries* 69, no. 7 (November 2020): 1–29, doi:10.15585/mmwr.ss6907a1.

Chapter 6

1. Christian Medical and Dental Associations, "Biblical Model for Medical Ethics," *CMDA Ethics Statements*, 2018, https://cmda.org/wp-content/uploads/2018/04/Biblical-Model-with-References.pdf.

2. Wendy Adele Humphrey, "'But I'm Brain-Dead and Pregnant': Advance Directive Pregnancy Exclusions and End-of-Life Wishes," *William & Mary Journal of Women and the Law* 21, no. 3 (2015): 669–98, https://scholarship.law.wm.edu/wmjowl/vol21/iss3/4.

3. Lauren Vogel, "Legal Storm Brewing over Texas Forced Life-Support Case," *Canadian Medical Association Journal* 186, no. 3 (2014): 107–8, https://www.ncbi.nlm.nih.gov/pmc/articles/PMC3928228/.

4. Vogel, "Legal Storm Brewing," 107–8.

5. Humphrey, "'Brain-Dead and Pregnant,'" 671.

6. Humphrey, "'Brain-Dead and Pregnant,'" 673.

7. Humphrey, "'Brain-Dead and Pregnant,'" 671.

8. Wikipedia, s.v. "Death of Marlise Muñoz," last modified July 22, 2021, 03:59. https://en.wikipedia.org/wiki/Death_of_Marlise_Muñoz.

9. Humphrey, "'Brain-Dead and Pregnant,'" 673.

10. Keith Moore, *Essentials of Human Embryology* (Toronto: B. C. Decker, 1988), 2. See also "When Does Life Begin . . . and End with EPC's," Issues and Action, United States Conference of Catholic Bishops, https://www.usccb.org/issues-and-action/human-life-and-dignity/abortion/when-does-life-begin-and-end-with-epcs.

11. Ronan O'Rahilly and Fabiola Müller, *Human Embryology and Teratology*, 2nd ed. (New York: Wiley-Liss, 1996), 29.

12. Stephen Napier, "Identifying Organism," *Linacre Quarterly* 84, no. 2 (2017): 151, https://www.ncbi.nlm.nih.gov/pmc/articles/PMC5499223/.

13. Napier, "Identifying Organism," 150.

14. Father James McTavish, "Suffering, Death, and Eternal Life," *The Linacre Quarterly* 83, no. 2 (2016): 134–41, https://www.ncbi.nlm.nih.gov/pmc/articles/PMC5102199/.

15. McTavish, "Suffering," 137–38.

16. McTavish, "Suffering," 138.

17. Neurocritical Care Society, "Brain Death: Frequently Asked Questions for the General Public," https://bioethics.yale.edu/sites/default/files/files/Brain%20Death%20FAQ%20-%20final%20posted.pdf.

18. Neurocritical Care Society, "Brain Death."

19. Vogel, "Legal Storm Brewing," 108.

20. Vogel, "Legal Storm Brewing," 108.

21. Napier, "Identifying Organism," 149.

22. Associated Press, "Purvi Patel is released after feticide conviction overturned," *IndyStar*, September 2, 2016, https://www.indystar.com/story/news/crime/2016/09/01/purvi-patel-releases-feticide-conviction-overturned/89707582/.

23. Associated Press, "Purvi Patel."

24. Charles C. Camosy, *Beyond the Abortion Wars* (Grand Rapids: Eerdmans, 2015).

25. Jennifer Hartline, "A Right to Not Be Pregnant? A Conflict of Interests," *The Stream*, January 26, 2020, https://stream.org/a-right-to-not-be-pregnant-a-conflict-of-interests/.

26. Judith Jarvis Thomson, "A Defense of Abortion," *Philosophy &*

Public Affairs 1, no. 1 (1971): 47–66, https://www.jstor.org/stable/2265091.

27. Sarah Zhang, "The Last Children of Down Syndrome," *The Atlantic*, November 18, 2020, https://www.theatlantic.com/magazine/archive/2020/12/the-last-children-of-down-syndrome/616928/.

Chapter 7

1. Institute of Medicine, *Dying in America: Improving Quality and Honoring Individual Preferences Near the End of Life* (Washington, DC: The National Academies Press, 2015).

2. Helen Taylor, "Legal Issues in End-of-Life Care 1: The Adult Patient," *Nursing Times* 114, no. 11 (2018): 25–28, https://www.nursingtimes.net/clinical-archive/end-of-life-and-palliative-care/legal-issues-in-end-of-life-care-1-the-adult-patient-15-10-2018/.

3. ANA Center for Ethics and Human Rights, "Nurses' Roles and Responsibilities in Providing Care and Support at the End of Life," *American Nurses Association*, 2016, https://www.nursingworld.org/~4af078/globalassets/docs/ana/ethics/endoflife-positionstatement.pdf.

4. Helen Taylor, "Legal Issues in End-of-Life Care 1: The Adult Patient," *Nursing Times*, 114, no. 11 (2018): 25–28, https://www.nursingtimes.net/clinical-archive/end-of-life-and-palliative-care/legal-issues-in-end-of-life-care-1-the-adult-patient-15-10-2018/.

5. Jim Woods, "Working with Dr. Husel at Mount Carmel Brought Trouble to Colleagues," *The Columbus Dispatch*, May 17, 2020, https://www.dispatch.com/news/20200517/working-with-dr-husel-at-mount-carmel-brought-trouble-to-colleagues.

6. Woods, "Dr. Husel."

7. Kantele Franko, "Ohio Hospital Reports 48 Nurses, Pharmacists Over Dosages, Deaths," *Insurance Journal*, March 15, 2020, https://www.insurancejournal.com/news/midwest/2019/03/15/520815.htm.

8. Franko, "Ohio Hospital."

9. Erik Ortiz, "Nurses Defend Ohio Doctor Accused of Murdering 25 Patients in Lawsuit against Hospital," *NBC News*, December 19, 2019, https://www.nbcnews.com/news/crime-courts/nurses

-defend-ohio-doctor-accused-murdering-25-patients-lawsuit -against-n1102796.

10. Robert D. Truog, Christine Mitchell, and George Q. Daley, "The Toughest Triage—Allocating Ventilators in a Pandemic," *The New England Journal of Medicine* 382 (2020): 1973–75, https://www.nejm.org /doi/full/10.1056/nejmp2005689.

11. Molly Olsen, Keith M. Swetz, and Paul S. Mueller, "Ethical Decision Making with End-of-Life Care: Palliative Sedation and Withholding or Withdrawing Life-Sustaining Treatments," *Mayo Clinic Proceedings* 85, no. 10 (2010): 949–54, https://www.ncbi.nlm.nih.gov /pmc/articles/PMC2947968/.

12. Human Rights Watch, "They Want Docile," February 2018, https://www.hrw.org/report/2018/02/05/they-want-docile/how -nursing-homes-united-states-overmedicate-people-dementia.

13. For more on this topic see chapter 7 of Charles C. Camosy, *Resisting Throwaway Culture: How a Consistent Life Ethic Can Unite a Fractured People* (New York: New City Press, 2019).

Chapter 8

1. Trisha Torrey, "Boutique Medicine and Concierge Practice," *VeryWell Health*, June 28, 2020, https://www.verywellhealth.com /what-is-boutique-medicine-a-concierge-doctor-practice-2615093.

2. "Welcome to Victors Care," Victors Care, https://www.victors care.org/.

3. Sumit Agarwal, "Physicians Who Refuse to Accept Medicaid Patients Breach Their Contract with Society," *Stat News*, December 28, 2017, https://www.statnews.com/2017/12/28/medicaid-physicians -social-contract/.

4. Winston R. Liaw et al., "Solo and Small Practices: A Vital, Diverse Part of Primary Care," *Annals of Family Medicine* 14, no. 1 (2016): 8–15, doi:10.1370/afm.1839.

5. Josiah Bates, "Ohio Began Mass Testing Incarcerated People for COVID-19. The Results Paint a Bleak Picture for the U.S. Prison

System," *Time*, April 22, 2020, https://time.com/5825030/ohio-mass-testing-prisons-coronavirus-outbreaks/.

6. "In-Prison Ministry," Prison Fellowship, last modified January 2021, https://www.prisonfellowship.org/resources/training-resources/in-prison/.

7. "National Nurse Practitioner Week: NPs Are Key to Providing Better Rural Care," *AANP News*, November 13, 2019, https://www.aanp.org/news-feed/national-nurse-practitioner-week-nps-are-key-to-providing-better-rural-care.

8. Teo Armus, "Nebraska Governor Says Citizens, Legal Residents Will Get Vaccine Priority over Undocumented Immigrants," *The Washington Post*, January 6, 2021, https://www.washingtonpost.com/nation/2021/01/06/nebraska-covid-vaccine-immigrants-meatpacking/.

9. This, of course, does not prohibit a nation having a clear and enforceable immigration policy—perhaps out of a gospel-centered concern to avoid its exploitation by those who want to hurt vulnerable immigrants via sex and other kinds of trafficking. But we are focused on the vocational commitments of Christian health-care providers, not immigration policy for particular countries. That latter topic is beyond the scope of this chapter.

10. "ICDC Complaint Letter," Project South, September 14, 2020, https://projectsouth.org/wp-content/uploads/2020/09/OIG-ICDC-Complaint-1.pdf.

11. José Olivares and John Washington, "A Silent Pandemic," *The Intercept*, September 14, 2020, https://theintercept.com/2020/09/14/ice-detention-center-nurse-whistleblower/.

12. Olivares and Washington, "Silent Pandemic."

13. Caitlin Dickerson, Seth Freed Wessler, and Miriam Jordan, "Immigrants Say They Were Pressured into Unneeded Surgeries," *New York Times*, September 29, 2020, https://www.nytimes.com/2020/09/29/us/ice-hysterectomies-surgeries-georgia.html.

14. Dickerson, Wessler, and Jordan, "Immigrants Say They Were Pressured."

15. Dickerson, Wessler, and Jordan, "Immigrants Say They Were Pressured."

16. Armus, "Nebraska Governor."

17. Dawn Wooten, "Nurse Speaks Out about 'Inhumane' Conditions at Georgia Immigrant Jail," *NBC News NOW*, September 16, 2020, YouTube Video, https://www.youtube.com/watch?v=RLZnoo_zBZk.

Chapter 9

1. Tedros Adhanom Ghebreyesus, "Health Is a Fundamental Human Right," *World Health Organization Newsroom*, December 10, 2017, https://www.who.int/news-room/commentaries/detail/health-is-a-fundamental-human-right#:~:text=The%2520right%2520to%2520health%2520for,them%252C%2520without%2520suffering%2520financial%2520hardship.&text=Discrimination%2520in%2520health%2520care%2520is,a%2520major%2520barrier%2520to%2520development.

2. D. L. Sansom, "Healthcare, Religious Obligations, and Caring for the Poor," *Ethics and Medicine* 35, no. 2 (2019): 117–26.

3. Matt Sedensky and Bernard Condon, "Not Just COVID: Nursing Home Neglect Deaths Surge in Shadows," *AP News*, November 19, 2020, https://apnews.com/article/nursing-homes-neglect-death-surge-3b74a2202140c5a6b5cf05cdf0ea4f32.

4. Tucker Doherty, "Summer Wave of Dementia Deaths Adds Thousands to Pandemic's Deadly Toll," *Politico*, September 16, 2020, https://www.politico.com/news/2020/09/16/dementia-deaths-coronavirus-nursing-homes-416530.

5. "Elder Abuse Facts," Public Policy & Action, National Council on Aging, https://www.ncoa.org/public-policy-action/elder-justice/elder-abuse-facts/.

6. Ethan Forman, "Nursing Home Found at Fault; Jury Issues $14.5M Verdict," *Newbury Port Daily News*, July 24, 2014, https://www.newburyportnews.com/news/local_news/nursing-home-found-at-fault-jury-issues-14-5m-verdict/article_886d2a2d-220d-598c-985e-b126f1825c90.html.

7. Irvin Jackson, "Massachusetts Nursing Home Lawsuit Results in $14M Verdict," *About Lawsuits*, July 29, 2014, https://www.about lawsuits.com/massachusetts-nursing-home-lawsuit-verdict-68500/.

8. Cappetta Law Office, "$14 Million Dollar Verdict in Middlesex County," *Massachusetts Personal Injury Blog*, July 23, 2014, https:// www.massachusettspersonalinjurylawyer-blog.com/14-million-dol lar-verdict-middlesex-county/.

9. Forman, "Nursing Home."

10. Forman, "Nursing Home."

11. Michael Specter, "The Dangerous Philosopher," *New Yorker*, September 6, 1999, http://archives.newyorker.com /?i=1999-09-06 #folio=CV1.

12. Here we want to highlight Charlie's recent book on this topic: Charles C. Camosy, *Losing Our Dignity: How Secularized Medicine Has Undermined Fundamental Human Equality* (Hyde Park, NY: New City Press, 2021).

13. "World Alzheimer Report 2015: The Global Impact of Dementia Summary Sheet," Alzheimer's Disease International, August 2015, https://www.alz.co.uk/research/WorldAlzheimerReport2015-sheet .pdf.

14. This is already happening in several places around the world, including the United Kingdom. Robert Booth, "Robots to Be Used in UK Care Homes to Help Reduce Loneliness," *The Guardian*, September 7, 2020, https://www.theguardian.com/society/2020 /sep/07/robots-used-uk-care-homes-help-reduce-loneliness?utm_ term=Autofeed&CMP=twt_gu&utm_medium&utm_source=Twit ter#Echobox=1599490685.

Chapter 10

1. Jennifer Blanchard, "Who Decides, Patient or Family?," *Virtual Mentor* 9, no. 8 (2007): 537–42, https://doi.org/10.1001/virtualmentor .2007.9.8.ccas3-0708.

2. Sumytra Menon, Vikki Entwistle, Alastair Campbell, and Jo-

hannes J. M. van Delden, "Some Unresolved Ethical Challenges in Healthcare Decision-Making: Navigating Family Involvement," *Asian Bioethics Review* 12 (2020): 27–36, https://link.springer.com/article/10.1007/s41649-020-00111-9.

3. "Why Withholding Information from Terminally Ill Patients Can Be a Good Thing," *Today's Hospitalist*, June 2005, https://www.todayshospitalist.com/Why-withholding-information-from-terminally-ill-patients-can-be-a-good-thing/.

4. M. D. Pérez-Cárceles, J. E. Pereñiguez, E. Osuna, and A. Luna, "Balancing Confidentiality and the Information Provided to Families of Patients in Primary Care," *Journal of Medical Ethics* 31, no. 9 (2005): 531–35, https://jme.bmj.com/content/31/9/531.

5. Brian Boyle, "The Critical Role of Family in Patient Experience," *Patient Experience Journal* 2, no. 2 (2015): 4–6, https://pxjournal.org/cgi/viewcontent.cgi?article=1112&context=journal. Rana Awdish, "Keeping Loved Ones from Visiting Our Coronavirus Patients Is Making Them Sicker," *The Washington Post*, August 6, 2020, https://www.washingtonpost.com/outlook/2020/08/06/coronavirus-icu-patients-families/.

Chapter 11

1. Kaya Oakes, "The 'Nones' Are Alright: What We Can Learn from a Generation of Seekers," *America Magazine*, 17 June, 2013, https://www.americamagazine.org/faith/2014/03/18/nones-are-alright-what-we-can-learn-generation-seekers.

2. Charles C. Camosy, "Study Shows Younger People Lack Faith in Religious Institutions," Interview by Josh Packard, *Crux*, February 17, 2021, https://cruxnow.com/interviews/2021/02/study-shows-younger-people-lack-faith-in-religious-institutions/.

3. Danish Zaidi, "Influences of Religion and Spirituality in Medicine," *AMA Journal of Ethics* 20, no. 7 (2018): 609–12, https://journalofethics.ama-assn.org/article/influences-religion-and-spirituality-medicine/2018-07.

4. April R. Christensen, Tara E. Cook, and Robert M. Arnold, "How Should Clinicians Respond to Requests from Patients to Participate in Prayer?," *AMA Journal of Ethics* 20, no. 7 (2018): 621–29, https://journalofethics.ama-assn.org/article/how-should-clinicians-respond-requests-patients-participate-prayer/2018-07.

5. Christensen, Cook, and Arnold, "Clinicians," 622.

6. Andrea C. Phelps, Michael T. Balboni, and Tracy A. Balboni, "Addressing Spirituality within the Care of Patients at the End of Life: Perspectives of Patients with Advanced Cancer, Oncologists, and Oncology Nurses," *Journal of Clinical Oncology* 30, no. 20 (2012): 2538–44, https://ascopubs.org/doi/10.1200/JCO.2011.40.3766.

7. Phelps, Balboni, and Balboni, "Addressing Spirituality," 2542.

8. Michael J. Balboni et al., "Why Is Spiritual Care Infrequent at the End of Life? Spiritual Care Perceptions among Patients, Nurses, and Physicians and the Role of Training," *Journal of Clinical Oncology* 31, no. 4 (2013): 461–67, https://ascopubs.org/doi/10.1200/JCO.2012.44.6443.

9. Stephen G. Post, "Physician and Patient Spirituality: Professional Boundaries, Competency, and Ethics," *Annals of Internal Medicine* 132, no. 7 (April 2000): 578, https://www.stephengpost.com/downloads/Stephen%20G.%20Post%20-%20Physicians%20and%20Patient%20Spirituality.pdf.

10. Post, "Physician and Patient Spirituality," 579.

11. Edgar A. Guest, "Sermons We See," *The Light*, March-April 1920, 44.

12. Martin Pengelly, "Nurse Who Treated Pittsburgh Shooter: 'I'm Sure He Had No Idea I Was Jewish,'" *The Guardian*, November 4, 2018, https://www.theguardian.com/us-news/2018/nov/04/pittsburgh-shooting-robert-bowers-jewish-nurse.

13. YeounSoo Kim-Godwin, "Prayer in Clinical Practice: What Does Evidence Support?" *Journal of Christian Nursing* 30, no. 4 (2013): 208–15, https://nursing.ceconnection.com/ovidfiles/00005217-201312000-00009.pdf.

14. Elizabeth Johnston Taylor, "Spiritual Care: Evangelism at the Bedside?" *Journal of Christian Nursing* 28, no. 4 (2018): 194–202, https://

journals.lww.com/journalofchristiannursing/Fulltext/2011/12000/Spiritual_Care__Evangelism_at_the_Bedside_.8.aspx.

15. "A Christian Nurse Suspended for Offering to Pray Has Sparked Health Care and Religion Debate," *Nursing Times*, February 24, 2009, https://www.nursingtimes.net/archive/a-christian-nurse-suspended-for-offering-to-pray-has-sparked-health-care-and-religion-debate-24-02-2009/.

16. "Christian Nurse Suspended."

17. Taylor, "Spiritual Care," 195.

18. Meg Hunter-Kilmer, "Let People Say of Us, 'See How They Love One Another!,'" *Aleteia*, June 19, 2016, https://aleteia.org/2016/06/19/let-people-say-of-us-see-how-they-love-each-other/.

19. Though it is worth noting that, in many cases, the lack of blood products makes little or no difference in the physical health outcomes. See Nicolas Jabbour, Singh Gagandeep, Rodrigo Mateo, Linda Sher, Earl Strum, John Donovan, Jeffrey Kahn, Christian G. Peyre, Randy Henderson, Tse-Ling Fong, Rick Selby, and Yuri Genyk, "Live Donor Liver Transplantation without Blood Products: Strategies Developed for Jehovah's Witnesses Offer Broad Application," *Annals of Surgery* 240, no. 2 (2004): 350–57, https://www.ncbi.nlm.nih.gov/pmc/articles/PMC1356413/.

Chapter 12

1. Second Vatican Council, "Pastoral Constitution on the Church in the Modern World *Gaudium et spes* Promulgated by His Holiness, Pope Paul VI on December 7, 1965," http://www.vatican.va/archive/hist_councils/ii_vatican_council/documents/vat-ii_cons_19651207_gaudium-et-spes_en.html.

2. Emma Green, "The Trump Administration Sides with Nurses Who Object to Abortion," *The Atlantic*, August 28, 2019, https://www.theatlantic.com/politics/archive/2019/08/nurse-abortion-against-will-vermont/596941/.

3. HHS Press Office, "OCR Issues Notice of Violation to the University of Vermont Medical Center after It Unlawfully Forced a Nurse

to Assist in Abortion," HHS, August 28, 2019, https://public3.pagefreezer.com/browse/HHS.gov/31-12-2020T08:51/https://www.hhs.gov/about/news/2019/08/28/ocr-issues-notice-violation-university-vermont-medical-center-after-it-unlawfully-forced-nurse.html.

4. ADF Staff, "NY Nurse Threatened, Forced to Assist in Late-Term Abortion," Alliance Defending Freedom, October 18, 2017, https://www.adflegal.org/press-release/ny-nurse-threatened-forced-assist-late-term-abortion.

5. ADF Staff, "NY Nurse Threatened."

6. "New York v. HHS," The Becket Fund for Religious Liberty, https://www.becketlaw.org/case/new-york-v-hhs/.

7. California Health and Safety Code, Sec. 123418, https://california.public.law/codes/ca_health_and_safety_code_section_123418.

8. Ian D. Wolfe and Thaddeus M. Pope, "Hospital Mergers and Conscience-Based Objections—Growing Threats to Access and Quality of Care," *The New England Journal of Medicine* 382, no. 15 (2020): 1388–89, https://www.nejm.org/doi/pdf/10.1056/NEJMp1917047?listPDF=true.

9. Wesley Smith, "California Bill to Force M.D. Participation in Assisted Suicide," *National Review*, February 11, 2021, https://www.nationalreview.com/corner/california-bill-to-force-m-d-participation-in-assisted-suicide/.

10. Wesley Smith, "Obliged to Kill," *Washington Examiner*, March 2, 2018, https://www.washingtonexaminer.com/weekly-standard/obliged-to-kill.

11. Ronit Y. Stahl and Ezekiel J. Emanuel, "Physicians, Not Conscripts—Conscientious Objection in Health Care," *New England Journal of Medicine* 376, no. 14 (2017): 1380–85, https://www.nejm.org/doi/full/10.1056/NEJMsb1612472.

12. Udo Schuklenk, "Professionalism Eliminates Religion as a Proper Tool for Doctors Rendering Advice to Patients," *Journal of Medical Ethics* 45, no. 11 (2019): 713, https://jme.bmj.com/content/45/11/713.

13. Rachel Browne, "Medical Schools Should Deny Applications Who Object to Provide Abortion, Assisted Death: Bioethicist," *Global News*, November 23, 2019, https://globalnews.ca/news/6183548/med

ical-school-applicants-abortion-assisted-death-conscientious-objectors/.

14. "California Defends Authority to Require Insurers to Cover Abortion as Protecting Women's Rights," *KHN Morning Briefing*, February 24, 2020, https://khn.org/morning-breakout/california-defends-authority-to-require-insurers-to-cover-abortion-as-protecting-womens-rights/.

15. United States Court of Appeals, Nos. 19-4254(L), 20–31, 20–32, 20–41, http://media.aclj.org/pdf/ACLJ-Amicus-brief-State-of-New-York-v.-HHS_Redacted.pdf.

16. "WMA Declaration on Euthanasia and Physician-Assisted Suicide," The World Medical Association, November 13, 2019, https://www.wma.net/policies-post/declaration-on-euthanasia-and-physician-assisted-suicide/.

17. AMA Staff, "Physicians Vote to Exercise Conscience in Medical Care," AMA, November 10, 2014, https://www.ama-assn.org/delivering-care/ethics/physicians-vote-exercise-conscience-medical-care.

18. 410 U.S. 179, 197–98 (1973).

19. "Conscience Protections for Health Care Providers," HHS, https://www.hhs.gov/conscience/conscience-protections/index.html.

20. "Life Matters: Conscience Protection in Health Care," United States Conference of Catholic Bishops, https://www.usccb.org/committees/religious-liberty/conscience-protection and https://www.usccb.org/committees/pro-life-activities/life-matters-conscience-protection-health-care.

21. Hannah Brockhaus, "Religious Freedom Is about Human Dignity, Pope Says in Morocco," *Catholic News Agency*, March 30, 2019, https://www.catholicnewsagency.com/news/religious-freedom-is-about-human-dignity-pope-says-in-morocco-19765.

22. Associated Press, "Pope Francis Says Conscientious Objection a 'Human Right,'" *Los Angeles Times*, September 28, 2015, 8:54 a.m. PT, https://www.latimes.com/nation/la-na-pope-visit-papal-plane-20150928-story.html.

23. Jill Waggoner, "ERLC Commends HHS Announcement of Final Rule Protecting Conscience Freedom in Healthcare," ERLC, May 3,

2019, https://erlc.com/resource-library/press-releases/erlc-commends-hhs-announcement-of-final-rule-protecting-conscience-freedom-in-healthcare/.

24. Waggoner, "ERLC Commends HHS Announcement."

25. Jonathan Imbody, "Intolerance of Conscience Threatens Diversity in Medicine," *CMDA's The Point* (blog), October 4, 2018, https://cmda.org/intolerance-of-conscience-threatens-diversity-in-medicine/.

26. Ezra Gabbay and Joseph Fins, "Go in Peace: Brain Death, Reasonable Accommodation and Jewish Mourning Rituals," *Journal of Religion and Health* 58 (2019): 1672–86, https://link.springer.com/article/10.1007/s10943-019-00874-y; and "Nursing with Dignity Part 1: Judaism," *Nursing Times* 98, no. 9 (2002): 35, https://www.nursingtimes.net/roles/nurse-managers/nursing-with-dignity-part-1-judaism-28-02-2002/.

27. Roni Caryn Rabin, "Respecting Muslim Patients' Needs," *New York Times*, November 1, 2010, https://www.nytimes.com/2010/11/01/health/01patients.html.

28. "Home," Secular Pro-Life Website, https://www.secularprolife.org/.

29. Care Quality Commission, *Review of Do Not Attempt Cardiopulmonary Resuscitation Decisions during the COVID-19 Pandemic*, November 2020, 34, https://www.cqc.org.uk/sites/default/files/20201204%20DNACPR%20Interim%20Report%20-%20FINAL.pdf.

30. Michael Cook, "UK Bureaucrats Imposed DNR Orders on Care Homes: Report," *BioEdge*, August 29, 2020, https://www.bioedge.org/mobile/view/uk-bureaucrats-imposed-dnr-orders-on-care-homes-report/13532.

31. "Major New Survey of Care Home Leaders Confirms Severe Impact of Covid-19," The Queen's Nursing Institute, August 24, 2020, https://www.qni.org.uk/news-and-events/news/major-new-survey-of-care-home-leaders-confirms-severe-impact-of-covid-19/.

Chapter 13

1. "Nursing and Midwifery," World Health Organization, May 2019, https://www.who.int/hrh/nursing_midwifery/en/.

2. "Healthcare Costs for Americans Projected to Grow at an Alarmingly High Rate," *Peter G. Peterson Foundation* (blog), May 1, 2019, https://www.pgpf.org/blog/2019/05/healthcare-costs-for-americans-projected-to-grow-at-an-alarmingly-high-rate.

3. A. Mund, "Healthcare Policy for Advocacy in Health Care," in *The Doctor of Nursing Practice Essentials*, ed. Mary Zaccagnini and Judith M. Pechacek (Burlington, MA: Jones & Bartlett Learning, 2019), 189–231.

4. J. W. Goldsberry, "Advanced Practice Nurses Leading the Way: Interprofessional Collaboration," *Nurse Education Today* 65 (2018): 1–3, https://doi.org/10.1016/j.nedt.2018.02.024.

5. Linda T. Kohn, Janet M. Corrigan, and Molla S. Donaldson, eds., *To Err Is Human: Building a Safer Health System* (Washington, DC: National Academies Press, 2000), doi:10.17226/9728.

6. Katherin J. Moran, Rosanne Berson, and Dianne Conrad, eds., *The Doctor of Nursing Practice Scholarly Project: A Framework for Success* (Burlington, MA: Jones & Bartlett Learning, 2017).

7. H. T. Stelfox, S. Palmisani, C. Scurlock, E. J. Oray, and D. W. Bates, "The 'To Err is Human' Report and Patient Safety Literature," *Quality and Safety in Healthcare* 15, no. 2 (June 2006): 174–78, https://doi.org/10.1136/qshc.2006.017947.

8. B. M. Melnyk and E. Fineout-Overholt, eds., *Evidence-Based Practice in Nursing and Healthcare: A Guide to Best Practice* (Philadelphia: Lippincott Williams & Wilkins, 2018), xviii–xxi.

9. S. A. Edwardson, "Imagining the DNP Role," in *The Doctor of Nursing Practice Essentials*, ed. Mary Zaccagnini and Judith M. Pechacek (Burlington, MA: Jones & Bartlett Learning, 2019), xvii–xxviii.

10. Susan E. Mazer, "Is Whole Person Care What Patients Want?," *Healing Healthcare Systems* (blog), January 2017, https://www.healinghealth.com/wp/whole-person-care-what-patients-want/.

11. M. B. Zeni, *Principles of Epidemiology for Advanced Nursing Practice: A Population Health Perspective* (Burlington, MA: Jones & Bartlett Learning, 2021).

12. Erin Westphal, "Managing Chronic Disease in an Evolving Healthcare Environment: Community-Based Organizations Increasingly Are Addressing Social Determinants of Health, and Preventing

More Expensive Medical Interventions," *Generations: Journal of the American Society on Ageing* 43, supplement 1 (2019): 4–7.

13. Goldsberry, "Advanced Practice Nurses," 1–3.

14. Michelle Clarke, "Nurses Have Potential to Transform Healthcare System, Says RWJF Report," *Health Leaders Media*, March 20, 2019, https://www.healthleadersmedia.com/nursing/nurses-have-potential-transform-healthcare-system-says-rwjf-report.

15. Goldsberry, "Advanced Practice Nurses," 1.

16. Laurel Ash, Catherine Miller, and Mary Zaccagnini, "Interprofessional Collaboration for Improving Patient and Population Health," in *The Doctor of Nursing Practice Essentials*, ed. Mary Zaccagnini and Kathryn White (Burlington, MA: Jones & Bartlett Learning, 2011), 233–74.

17. Ash, Miller, and Zaccagnini, "Interprofessional Collaboration," 239.

18. Daniel Weberg, "Innovation Leadership Behaviors: Starting the Complexity Journey," in *Leadership for Evidence-Based Innovation in Nursing and Health Professions*, ed. Sandra Davidson, Daniel Weberg, Tim Porter-O'Grady, and Kathy Malloch (Burlington, MA: Jones & Bartlett Learning, 2019), 43–76.

19. Rebecca Patton and Margaret Zalon, "Leading the Way in Policy," in *Nurses Making Policy: From Bedside to Boardroom*, ed. Ruth Ludwick, Rebecca Patton, and Margaret Zalon (New York: Springer, 2014), 3–39.

20. Mary Davenport, Jennifer Lahl, and Evan Rosa, "Right of Conscience for Healthcare Providers," *Linacre Quarterly* 79, no. 2 (May 2012): 169–91, https://doi.org/10.1179/002436312803571357.

21. Davenport, Lahl, and Rosa, "Right of Conscience," 175.

22. Davenport, Lahl, and Rosa, "Right of Conscience," 179.

23. Charles C. Camosy, *Losing Our Dignity: How Secularized Medicine Has Undermined Fundamental Human Equality* (Hyde Park, NY: New City Press, 2021).

24. Aimee Milliken, "Ethical Awareness: What It Is and Why It Matters," *The Online Journal of Issues in Nursing* 23, no. 1 (2018), https://ojin.nursingworld.org/MainMenuCategories/ANAMarket

place/ANAPeriodicals/OJIN/TableofContents/Vol-23-2018/No1-Jan-2018/Ethical-Awareness.html.

Chapter 14

1. Edmund Lee, "Nurses Share Coronavirus Stories Anonymously in an Online Document," *New York Times*, March 25, 2020, https://www.nytimes.com/2020/03/25/business/media/coronavirus-nurses-stories-anonymous.html.

2. This conversation was conducted in confidentiality, and the nurse's name is withheld by mutual consent.

3. https://nurses.dearworld.org/.

4. https://nurses.dearworld.org/.

5. Patricia Nayna Scwedtle, Clifford Connell, Susan Lee, Virginia Plummer, Philip Russo, Ruth Endecott, and Lisa Kuhn, "Nurse Expertise: A Critical Resource in the COVID-19 Pandemic Response," *Annals of Global Health* 86, no. 1 (2020): 49, https://doi.org/10.5334/aogh.2898.

6. Scwedtle et al., "Nurse Expertise," 49.

7. Scwedtle et al., "Nurse Expertise," 49.

8. Megan Ford, "Even More Nurses Considering Quitting the Profession," *Nursing Times*, July 17, 2020, https://www.nursingtimes.net/news/workforce/even-more-nurses-considering-quitting-the-profession-survey-reveals-17-07-2020/.

9. "Supply and Demand Projections of the Nursing Workforce: 2014–2030," US Department of Health and Human Services, Health Resources and Services, Bureau of Health Workforce, and Center for Health Workforce Analysis, July 21, 2017, https://bhw.hrsa.gov/sites/default/files/bureau-health-workforce/data-research/nchwa-hrsa-nursing-report.pdf. See also Lisa Haddad, Pavan Annamaraju, and Tammy Toney-Butler, "Nursing Shortage," in *StatPearls* (Treasure Island, FL: StatPearls Publishing, 2021), https://www.ncbi.nlm.nih.gov/books/NBK493175/.

10. This conversation was conducted in confidentiality, and the nurse's name is withheld by mutual consent.

11. Amanda Bucceri Andros, "The (Not So) Great Escape: Why

Nurses Are Leaving the Profession," *Registered Nursing*, January 29, 2021, https://www.registerednursing.org/articles/why-new-nurses-leaving-profession/.

12. Ira John Sites, "Nurses Are Only Seen as Replaceable Numbers," *Nurse Jessica Sites* (blog), November 2, 2020, https://nursejessicasites.com/?p=809&fbclid=IwAR31iyVNL6LpPbTvUgSHJLq2RsvIeDCMCbHe8voQZ8xhrJKLSRrxPM7Qtyg.

13. Agustina Zaka, Soraya Shamloo, Pasquale Fiorente, and Alessandro Tafuri, "COVID-19 Pandemic as a Watershed Moment: A Call for Systematic Psychological Healthcare for Frontline Medical Staff," *Journal of Health Psychology* 27, no. 7 (2020): 883–87, https://doi.org/10.1177/1359105320925148. See also Julia Lynch, Nicholas Evans, Erin Ice, and Deena Kelly Costa, "Ignoring Nurses: Media Coverage during the COVID-19 Pandemic," *Annals of the American Thoracic Society* 18, no. 8 (2021): 1278–82, https://doi.org/10.1513/AnnalsATS.202010-1293PS.

14. Here it is worth recalling that many nuns were working with the elderly and disabled in the context of the COVID-19 pandemic, carrying on the tradition of women religious doing this throughout the centuries. See Emma Green, "Nuns vs. the Coronavirus," *The Atlantic*, May 3, 2020, https://www.theatlantic.com/politics/archive/2020/05/coronavirus-nursing-home-deaths/611053/.

FURTHER READING

HISTORY OF NURSING

Kelly, Mary P. "Hospital Nuns: From the Civil War to Today." *Irish America*, September 18, 2018. https://irishamerica.com/2013/08/hospital-nuns-from-the-civil-war-to-today/.

Koenig, Harold G. "Religion and Medicine I: Historical Background and Reasons for Separation." *International Journal of Psychiatry in Medicine* 30, no. 4 (December 2000): 385–98. http://citeseerx.ist.psu.edu/viewdoc/download?doi=10.1.1.521.9908&rep=rep1&type=pdf.

Levin, Peter J. "Bold Vision: Catholic Sisters and the Creation of American Hospitals." *Journal of Community Health* 36 (2011): 343–47. https://doi.org/10.1007/s10900-011-9401-7.

Sullivan, Mary C., ed. *The Friendship of Florence Nightingale and Mary Clare Moore*. Philadelphia: University of Pennsylvania Press, 1999.

Wall, B. M. "Definite Lines of Influence: Catholic Sisters and Nurse Training Schools, 1890–1920." *Nursing Research* 50, no. 5 (September/October 2001): 314–21. https://doi.org/10.1097/00006199-200109000-00010.

MEDICAL EUGENICS

Berghs, M., B. Dierckx de Casterlé, and C. Gastmans. "Nursing, Obedience, and Complicity with Eugenics: A Contextual Interpretation of Nursing Morality at the Turn of the Twentieth Century." *Journal of Medical Ethics* 32, no. 2 (2006): 117–22. https://doi.org/10.1136/jme.2004.011171.

Evans, Richard J. *The Third Reich at War.* New York: Penguin, 2009.

Farla, Audrey. "The Revival of Raced-Based Medicine: Eugenics, Religion, and the Black Experience." Review of *Medical Stigmata*, by K. A. Johnson. Marginalia. *Los Angeles Review of Books.* October 18, 2019. https://marginalia.lareviewofbooks.org/revival-of-raced-based-medicine-eugenics-religion-and-the-black-experience/.

Neugebauer, Wolfgang. "The Nazi Mass Murder of the Intellectually and the Physically Disabled and the Resistance of Sister Anna Bertha Königsegg." Lecture, Documentation Archive of the Austrian Resistance, Goldegg Castle, November 12, 1998.

Pius XI, Pope. *Casti Connubii.* December 31, 1930. https://w2.vatican.va/content/pius-xi/en/encyclicals/documents/hf_p-xi_enc_19301231_casti-connubii.html.

WHEN DOES LIFE BEGIN AND END?

Moore, Keith. *Essentials of Human Embryology.* Toronto: B. C. Decker, 1988.

Napier, Stephen. "Identifying Organism." *Linacre Quarterly* 84, no. 2 (2017): 145–54. https://www.ncbi.nlm.nih.gov/pmc/articles/PMC5499223/.

O'Rahilly, Ronan, and Fabiola Müller. *Human Embryology and Teratology.* 2nd ed. New York: Wiley-Liss, 1996.

United States Conference of Catholic Bishops. "When Does Life Begin . . . and End with EPC's." Issues and Action. Accessed October 4, 2021. https://www.usccb.org/issues-and-action/human-life-and-dignity/abortion/when-does-life-begin-and-end-with-epcs.

RESOURCE ALLOCATION IN NURSING

Falk, N. L., and E. S. Chong. "Beyond the Bedside: Nurses, a Critical Force in the Macroallocation of Resources." *OJIN: The Online*

Journal of Issues in Nursing 13, no. 2 (2008). https://doi.org/10.3912/OJIN.Vol13No02PPT01.

Kalisch, B. J., G. Landstrom, and A. Hinshaw. "Missed Nursing Care: A Concept Analysis." *Journal of Advanced Nursing* 67, no. 7 (2009): 1509–17.

Lee, Meina, and Elizabeth Geelhoed. "Teaching Resource Allocation—and Why It Matters." *AMA Journal of Ethics* 13, no. 4 (2011): 224–27. https://doi.org/10.1001/virtualmentor.2011.13.4.medu1-1104.

Scott, Anne, Clare Harvey, Heike Felzmann, Riitta Suhonen, Monika Habermann, Kristin Halvorsen, Karin Christiansen, Luisa Toffoli, and Evridiki Papastavrou. "Resource Allocation and Rationing in Nursing Care: A Discussion Paper." *Nursing Ethics* 26, no. 5 (2019): 1528–39. https://doi.org/10.1177/0969733018759831.

WHOLE-PERSON CARE

Goldsbery, J. W. "Advanced Practice Nurses Leading the Way: Interprofessional Collaboration." *Nurse Education Today* 65 (2018): 1–3. https://doi.org/10.1016/j.nedt.2018.02.024.

Mazer, Susan E. "Is Whole Person Care What Patients Want?" *Healing Healthcare Systems* (blog). January 2017. https://www.healinghealth.com/wp/whole-person-care-what-patients-want/.

Westphal, Erin. "Managing Chronic Disease in an Evolving Healthcare Environment: Community-Based Organizations Increasingly Are Addressing Social Determinants of Health, and Preventing More Expensive Medical Interventions." *Generations: Journal of the American Society on Ageing* (2019): 4–7.

PROTECTING CONSCIENCE IN MEDICINE AND NURSING

Davenport, Mary, Jennifer Lahl, and Evan Rosa. "Right of Conscience for Healthcare Providers." *Linacre Quarterly* 79, no. 2 (May 2012): 169–91. https://doi.org/10.1179/002436312803571357.

Imbody, Jonathan. "Intolerance of Conscience Threatens Diversity in Medicine." *CMDA's The Point* (blog). October 4, 2018. https://

cmda.org/intolerance-of-conscience-threatens-diversity-in-medicine/.

Stahl, Ronit Y., and Ezekiel J. Emanuel. "Physicians, Not Conscripts—Conscientious Objection in Health Care." *New England Journal of Medicine* 376, no. 14 (2017): 1380–85. https://doi.org/10.1056/NEJMsb1612472.

United States Conference of Catholic Bishops. "Conscience Protection." Accessed October 4, 2021. https://www.usccb.org/committees/religious-liberty/conscience-protection.

———. "Life Matters: Conscience Protection in Health Care." Accessed October 4, 2021. https://www.usccb.org/committees/pro-life-activities/life-matters-conscience-protection-health-care.

Wolfe, D., and Thaddeus M. Pope. "Hospital Mergers and Conscience-Based Objections — Growing Threats to Access and Quality of Care." *New England Journal of Medicine* 382, no. 15 (2020): 1388–89. https://doi.org/10.1056/NEJMp1917047.

HEALTHCARE DECISION-MAKING

Blanchard, Jennifer. "Who Decides, Patient or Family?" *Virtual Mentor: AMA Journal of Ethics* 9, no. 8 (2007): 537–42. https://doi.org/10.1001/virtualmentor.2007.9.8.ccas3-0708.

Boyle, Brian. "The Critical Role of Family in Patient Experience." *Patient Experience Journal* 2, no. 2 (2015): 4–6. https://pxjournal.org/cgi/viewcontent.cgi?article=1112&context=journal.

Menon, Sumytra, Vikki Entwistle, Alastair Campbell, and Johannes J. M. van Delden. "Some Unresolved Ethical Challenges in Healthcare Decision-Making: Navigating Family Involvement." *Asian Bioethics Review* 12 (2020): 27–36. https://doi.org/10.1007/s41649-020-00111-9.

Pérez-Cárceles, M. D., J. E. Pereñiguez, E. Osuna, and A. Luna. "Balancing Confidentiality and the Information Provided to Families of Patients in Primary Care." *Journal of Medical Ethics* 31, no. 9 (2005): 531–35.

NURSING ETHICS

Camosy, Charles C. *Losing Our Dignity: How Secularized Medicine Is Undermining Fundamental Human Equality.* Hyde Park, NY: New City Press, 2021.

Melnyk, B. M., and E. Fineout-Overholt, eds. *Evidence-Based Practice in Nursing and Healthcare: A Guide to Best Practice.* Philadelphia: Lippincott Williams & Wilkins, 2018.

Milliken, Aimee. "Ethical Awareness: What It Is and Why It Matters." *Online Journal of Issues in Nursing* 23, no. 1 (2018). https://doi.org/10.3912/OJIN.Vol23No01Man01.

GERIATRIC, ELDER, AND END-OF-LIFE CARE

ANA Center for Ethics and Human Rights. "Nurses' Roles and Responsibilities in Providing Care and Support at the End of Life." American Nurses Association. 2016. https://www.nursingworld.org/~4af078/globalassets/docs/ana/ethics/endoflife-positionstatement.pdf.

Congregation for the Doctrine of the Faith. *Samaritanus Bonus: On the Care of Persons in the Critical and Terminal Phases of Life.* November 21, 1964. http://www.vatican.va/roman_curia/congregations/cfaith/documents/rc_con_cfaith_doc_20200714_samaritanus-bonus_en.html.

Phelps, Andrea C., Michael T. Balboni, and Tracy A. Balboni. "Addressing Spirituality within the Care of Patients at the End of Life: Perspectives of Patients with Advanced Cancer, Oncologists, and Oncology Nurses." *Journal of Clinical Oncology* 30, no. 20 (2012): 2538–44.

Taylor, Helen. "Legal Issues in End-of-Life Care 1: The Adult Patient." *Nursing Times* 114, no. 11 (2018): 25–28.

SPIRITUALITY AND SPIRITUAL CARE IN NURSING CARE

Christensen, April R., Tara E. Cook, and Robert M. Arnold. "How Should Clinicians Respond to Requests from Patients to Participate in Prayer?" *AMA Journal of Ethics* 20, no. 7 (2018): 621–29.
Ellis, Ariana. "Healing Body and Spirit." *AMA Journal of Ethics* 20, no. 7 (2018): 668–69. https://doi.org/10.1001/amajethics.2018.668.
Kim-Godwin, YeounSoo. "Prayer in Clinical Practice: What Does Evidence Support?" *Journal of Christian Nursing* 30, no. 4 (2015): 2018–215. https://nursing.ceconnection.com/ovidfiles/00005217-201312000-00009.pdf.
Meehan, Therese. "Spirituality and Spiritual Care from a Careful Nursing Perspective." *Journal of Nursing Management* 20, no. 8 (2012): 990–10001. https://doi.org/10.1111/j.1365-2834.2012.01462.x.
O'Brien, Mary Elizabeth. *Spirituality in Nursing: Standing on Holy Ground.* 6th ed. Burlington, MA: Jones & Bartlett Learning, 2018.
Sansom, D. L. "Healthcare, Religious Obligations, and Caring for the Poor." *Ethics and Medicine* 35, no. 2 (2019): 117–26.
Zaidi, Danish. "Influences of Religion and Spirituality in Medicine." *AMA Journal of Ethics* 20, no. 7 (2018): 609–12. https://doi.org/10.1001/amajethics.2018.609.

CHRISTIAN ETHICS

Camosy, Charles C. *Beyond the Abortion Wars.* Grand Rapids: Eerdmans, 2015.
———. *Resisting Throwaway Culture: How a Consistent Life Ethic Can Unite a Fractured People.* New York: New City Press, 2019.
Curan, Charles. "The Catholic Moral Tradition in Bioethics." In *The*

Story of Bioethics: from Seminal Works to Contemporary Explorations, 113–29. Washington, DC: Georgetown University Press, 2003.

Kilner, John F. "The Bible, Ethics, and Health Care: Theological Foundations for a Christian Perspective on Health Care." CACE Ethics Booklets. 1992. https://www.wheaton.edu/media/migrated-images-amp-files/media/files/centers-and-institutes/cace/booklets/BibleEthicsHealthcare.pdf.

CHRISTIAN NURSING

Dameron, Carrie. "What Is the Essence of Christian Nursing?" *Journal of Christian Nursing* 27, no. 4 (October-December 2010): 285. https://doi.org/10.1097/CNJ.0b013e3181ee77d5.

Levin, Peter J. "Bold Vision: Catholic Sisters and the Creation of American Hospitals." *Journal of Community Health* 36 (2011): 343–47. https://doi.org/10.1007/s10900-011-9401-7.

Shelly, Judith Allen. *Called to Care: A Christian Worldview for Nursing*. Downers Grove, IL: IVP Academic, 2006.

INDEX